Chinese Fast Wrestling
for
Fighting

Chinese Fast Wrestling for Fighting

for

Fighting

The Art of
San Shou Kuai Jiao

Liang, Shou-Yu
&
Tai D. Ngo

YMAA Publication Center
Jamaica Plain, Mass. USA

YMAA Publication Center
Main Office:
    4354 Washington Street
    Roslindale, Massachusetts, 02130
    1-800-669-8892 • www.ymaa.com • ymaa@aol.com

10 9 8 7

Publisher's Cataloging in Publication
(Prepared by Quality Books Inc.)

Liang, Shou-Yu, 1943-
    Chinese fast wrestling for fighting : the art of San Shou Kuai
Jiao / Liang Shou-Yu and Tai D. Ngo.
      p. cm.
      Includes index.
      ISBN: 1-886969-49-3

      1. Martial arts—China. 2. Wrestling—China. I. Ngo, Tai D.
II. Title.

GV1100.7.A2L53 1997   796.8'0951
                              QBI97-40077

Disclaimer:
The authors and publisher of this material are NOT RESPONSIBLE in any manner whatsoever for any injury which may occur through reading or following the instructions in this manual.
The activities, physical or otherwise, described in this material may be too strenuous or dangerous for some people, and the reader(s) should consult a physician before engaging in them.

Printed in Canada.

A NOTE ON ENGLISH SPELLINGS OF CHINESE WORDS

YMAA Publication Center uses the Pinyin romanization system of Chinese to English. Pinyin is standard in the People's Republic of China, and in several world organizations, including the United Nations. Pinyin, which was introduced in China in the 1950's, replaces the Kwoyeu Romatzyh, Wade-Giles, and Yale systems.

SOME COMMON CONVERSIONS:

Kwoyeu Romatzyh	Pinyin	Pronunciation
Chi	Qi	Chee
Chi Kung	Qigong	Chee Kung
Chin Na	Qin Na	Chin Na
Jing	Jin	Jin
Kung Fu	Gongfu	Gong Foo
Tai Chi Chuan	Taijiquan	Tai Jee Chuen

For more complete conversion tables, please refer to the *People's Republic of China: Administrative Atlas,* the *Reform of the Chinese Written Language,* or a contemporary manual of style.

ACKNOWLEDGMENTS

Thanks to Dr. Yang, Jwing-Ming for encouragement, technical advice, and support. Thanks to Sam Masich and Huen Siu Hung for their time and effort. Thanks to Richard Rossiter for the cover design. Special thanks to Al Arsenault for writing and demonstrating the techniques in chapter 8. Thanks to Tim Comrie for his photography, Al Loriaux for his help in the last chapter and many YMAA members for general assistance, including Jeff Pratt, Kain Sanderson, Erik Elsemans, and June-Marie Mahay for proofreading. Thanks to Mei-Ling Yang for checking the Chinese translations. Also thanks to Andrew Murray for editing.

ABOUT THE AUTHOR

Master Liang, Shou-Yu 梁守渝

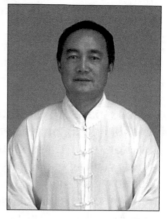

Master Liang, Shou-Yu was born on June 28, 1943 in the city of Chongqian, Sichuan Province (四川、重慶), China. When he was six he began his training in Qigong, the art of breathing and internal energy control, under the tutelage of his renowned grandfather, the late Liang, Zhi-Xiang (梁芷箱). Mr. Liang was taught the esoteric skills of the Emei Mountain sect, including Da Peng Qigong (大鵬氣功). When he was eight, his grandfather made special arrangements for him to begin training Emei Wushu (martial arts) (峨嵋武術).

In 1959, Mr. Liang began the study of Qin Na (擒拿) and Chinese Shuai Jiao (Wrestling) (摔跤). From 1960 to 1964 he devoted his attention to the systematic research and practice of Wrestling, Wushu, and other special martial power training.

In addition to the advantage of being born to a Wushu family, Mr. Liang also had the chance to come into contact with many legendary grandmasters. By the time he was twenty, Mr. Liang had already received instruction from 10 of the most well-known contemporary masters of both Southern and Northern origin, who gladly instructed and inspired this ardent young man. His curiosity inspired him to learn more than one hundred sequences from many different styles. His study of the martial arts has taken him throughout mainland China, having gone to Henan Province (河南) to learn Chen style Taijiquan, Hubei Province to learn the Wudang system, and Hubei Province (湖北) to learn the Nan Yue system.

With his wealth of knowledge, Mr. Liang was inspired to compete in martial arts competitions, in which he was many times a gold medalist in China. During his adolescence, Mr. Liang won titles in Chinese wrestling (Shuai Jiao), various other martial arts, and weight lifting.

Through and beyond his college years, Mr. Liang's wide background in various martial arts helped form his present character, and led him to achieve a high level of martial skill. Some of the styles he concentrated on include the esoteric Emei system, Shaolin Long Fist (少林長拳), Praying Mantis (螳螂), Chuo Jiao (戳腳), Xingyi (形意), Baguazhang (八卦掌), Taijiquan (太極拳), Liu He Ba Fa (六合八法), Shuai Jiao (摔跤), Qin Na (擒拿), vital point striking, many weapons systems, and several kinds of internal Qigong.

Mr. Liang received a university degree in biology and physiology from West-South National University in 1964. However, it was a time of political turmoil, and because of his bourgeois family background, the Communist government sent him to a remote, poverty-stricken area to teach high school. Despite this setback, Mr. Liang began to organize Wushu teams in the local community, and he trained numerous farmer-students in Wushu and in wrestling.

Then came a disastrous time in modern Chinese history. During the years of the Cultural Revolution (1966-1974 A.D.), all forms of martial arts and Qigong were suppressed. Because he came from a bourgeoisie family, Mr. Liang was vulnerable to the furious passions and blind madness of the revolutionaries. To avoid conflict with the Red Guards, he gave up his teaching position. Mr. Liang used this opportunity to tour various parts of the country to discover and visit great masters in Wushu, and to make friends with people who shared his devotion to and love for the art. Mr. Liang went through numerous provinces and large cities, visiting especially the many renowned and revered places where Wushu was created, developed, and polished. Among the many places he visited were Emei Mountain (峨嵋山), Wudang Mountain (武當山), Hua Mountain (華山), Qingchen Mountain (青城山), Chen's village in Henan (河南), the Cangzhou Territory (滄州) in Hebei Province (河北), Beijing (北京), and Shanghai (上海). In eight years he made many Wushu friends and met many great masters, and his mastery of the techniques and philosophy of the art grew to new horizons.

At the end of the Cultural Revolution, the Chinese government again began to support the martial arts and Qigong, including competitions. There was a general movement to organize and categorize the existing martial and internal arts. Research projects were set up to search out the old masters who remained alive, select their best techniques, and organize their knowledge. It was at this time that the Sichuan government appointed Mr. Liang as a coach for the city, the territory, and the province. So many of his students were among the top martial artists of China that in 1978 Mr. Liang was voted one of the top national coaches since 1949. He also received acclaim from the People's Republic of China Physical Education and Sports Commissions, and often served as judge in national competitions.

After the Cultural Revolution, and despite his many official duties, Mr. Liang continued to participate actively in competitions at the provincial and national level. Between 1974 and 1981 he won numerous medals, including four gold medals. His students also performed superbly in national and provincial open tournaments, winning many medals. Many of these students have now become professional Wushu coaches or college Wushu instructors themselves. Other students have become Wushu trainers in the armed forces, or have become movie actors in Wushu pictures. In 1979, Mr. Liang received several appointments, including a committee membership in the Sichuan Chapter of the China National Wushu Association, and an executive membership of the Wushu Coaches Committee.

1981 marked a new era in the course of Mr. Liang's life, when he first visited Seattle, Washington in the United States. His art impressed every one of the Wushu devotees immediately, and the Wushu and Taiji Club of the University of Washington retained him as a Wushu Coach. In addition, Mr. Liang offered lessons at the Taiji Association in Seattle. The following year, Mr. Liang went north to Vancouver, Canada, where he was appointed Taiji Coach by the Villa Cathy Care Home, and Honorary

Chairman and Head Coach by the North American Taiji Athletic Association.

In 1984, Mr. Liang became Chairperson and Wushu Coach for the School of Physical Education of the University of British Columbia. In 1985, he was elected coach of the First Canadian National Wushu Team, which was invited to participate in the First International Wushu Invitational Tournament in Xian, China. Competing against teams from 13 other countries, the Canadian team won third place.

In 1986, Mr. Liang was again elected coach of the Second Canadian National Wushu Team, which competed in the Second International Wushu Invitational Tournament held in the city of Teinstin, China. This time, 28 countries participated, and the Canadian team earned more medals than any other country except the host country itself. Mr. Liang's role and achievements were reported in 14 newspapers and magazines throughout China, and the performances and demonstrations of Mr. Liang and his team were broadcast on the Sichuan television station.

Mr. Liang has not limited his Wushu contributions to Canada. He has given numerous lectures and demonstrations to Wushu professionals and instructors in the United States. Adherents of many disciplines, including Karate, Taiji and others, have benefited from Mr. Liang's personal touch. In addition to instructing in such cities as Houston, Denver, Boston, and New York, Mr. Liang was invited to several cities in Italy for seminars in 1991. Mr. Liang has also judged in the National Wushu Tournament in the United States, and has produced an instructional video program teaching Liangong Shr Ba Fa Qigong (練功十八法) in conjunction with the Chinese National Qigong Institute.

ABOUT THE AUTHOR

Mr. Tai D. Ngo

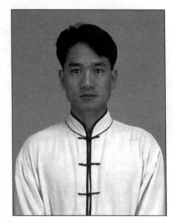

Tai D. Ngo was born in Viet Nam. In his adolescence he lived and traveled to various regions in Viet Nam and China, and became fluent in both languages. In 1981 Mr. Ngo came to Boston for school. In 1985, while at Northeastern University studying Electrical Engineering, Mr. Ngo began his martial arts training at Yang's Martial Arts Association (YMAA). Under the guidance of Dr. Yang, Jwing-Ming, Mr. Ngo learned Shaolin Long Fist and Shaolin White Crane Gongfu and Yang style Taijiquan.

After graduating from Northeastern University in 1988, Mr. Ngo went to work in the field of computers, and continued to train with Dr. Yang, eventually attaining the rank of Assistant Instructor. He then began to teach Shaolin and Taijiquan at YMAA Headquarters in Boston. In 1989, Mr. Ngo met Master Liang, Shou-Yu and learned Hsing Yi, Baguazhang, Chen style Taijiquan and was introduced to San Shou Kuai Jiao.

Since 1991, Mr. Ngo has been a top competitor in national martial arts tournaments in the United States. In 1992 he won the Men's All-Around Internal Styles Grand Champion at the United States National Chinese Martial Arts Competition in Orlando, Florida. In the same year he finished top in all the events he competed in at the United States Koushu Championship in Towson, Maryland. Also in the same year, Mr. Ngo was invited to join the United States Chinese Koushu National Team, and competed in the 7th World Koushu Tournament in Taiwan.

In 1994, Mr. Ngo won two gold medals for excellent performances in the World Grand Wushu Festival, the "Oberon Cup," held in Shanghai, China. He also toured and performed in many cities and towns in China with the North American Martial Arts Team, led by Master Liang. After returning from China, Mr. Ngo again won the Men's Internal Styles Grand Championship at the United States National Chinese Martial Arts Competition in Orlando, Florida.

Mr. Ngo continues to teach and train under Dr. Yang at YMAA Headquarters. He lives in Malden, Massachusetts. This is his first book.

FOREWORD

Dr. Yang, Jwing-Ming

It is commonly known in Chinese martial arts society that in order to fight effectively and survive in a battle, any proficient martial artist must acquire four basic categories of fighting techniques: kicking (Ti, 踢), punching (Da, 打), wrestling (Shuai, 摔), and Qin Na (Na, 拿). Technically speaking, wrestling was designed to deal with kicking and punching, Qin Na (i.e., joint control) was created to cope with wrestling, and kicking and punching were to be used against Qin Na. You can see that these four categories mutually support and also conquer each other. That means in order to become a proficient martial artist, you must master these four categories, which exist in every Chinese martial style.

When Chinese martial arts were imported to Japan, kicking and punching became Karate (空手道, The Dao of Barehand), wrestling became the root of Judo (柔道, The Dao of Softness), and Qin Na built the foundation of Jujitsu (柔術道, The Dao of Soft Techniques). Later, the combination of Judo and Jujitsu became today's Aikido (合氣道, The Dao of Harmonizing Qi).

For example, it is commonly recognized in Japanese Karate society that the root of Japanese Karate was Okinawan Karate, and Okinawan Karate originated from the Chinese Southern White Crane style of Fujian province, China. Not only that, it is recorded in Japanese documents, **Collection of Ancestor's Conversations** (先哲叢談), **Volume 2, Biography of Chen, Yuan-Yun** (卷二・陳元贇傳) that Chen, Yuan-Yun (1587-1671 A.D., Ming dynasty) was the person who brought the "soft techniques" (i.e., wrestling) into Japan in 1659 that became today's Judo.

When Chinese martial arts were imported to the West in the 1960's, the majority of techniques focused on kicking and punching. In order to make the contents of Western Chinese martial arts training more complete, I have written four Qin Na books to introduce the art of seizing and controlling. However, the Chinese wrestling arts are still not well-known or understood by Western Chinese martial artists. In order to fill this gap, I have been encouraging Master Liang to write a few books about Chinese wrestling. Master Liang is well known as an expert in this field, and he has won several gold medals in wrestling in China.

I am very happy to see that with Mr. Tai D. Ngo's help, this wrestling book is finally available to Western martial artists. In order to preserve the martial arts that have been developed over thousands of years of human history, we must put what we still know into books and on video. This way these arts will not become lost treasures.

Dr. Yang, Jwing-Ming
June 11, 1996

PREFACE

Master Liang, Shou-Yu

Traditional Chinese free fighting is generally called San Shou (散手). San Shou fighting includes the four main fighting categories of Ti (Kicking, 踢), Da (Striking, 打), Shuai (Wrestling, 摔), and Na (Qin Na, 擒拿). Among these four basic techniques, Shuai Jiao (Shuai) has an important value in San Shou fighting. In the past, winning a San Shou match required knocking your opponent off the Lei Tai (competition platform, 擂臺) or taking him down to the ground by using the skills of Ti, Da, Shuai, and Na. Therefore, Shuai Jiao is a very important skill when a martial artist is in a real combat situation. If a fighter does not have any Shuai Jiao experience or training, the chance of winning or surviving in a San Shou match is very slim. Therefore, more and more San Shou practitioners around the world are recognizing the combat value of Shuai Jiao and incorporating the techniques into their fighting styles. Even in daily life, Shuai Jiao can be an effective tool for self-defense. Combining the Shuai Jiao skill with your own self-defense skills can be a helpful weapon to fight off an attacker on the street. Because of its practical value, Shuai Jiao is an important part of Chinese martial arts.

All the different styles of Chinese Gongfu (功夫)(Wushu, 武術), have some Shuai Jiao training methods in their forms. Unfortunately, not all martial practitioner realize that there are Shuai Jiao techniques in their style. I believe this is because in traditional Gongfu training, a teacher will spend years to watch and test a student's morality to see if that student is worthy of teaching to pass on the secrets of their style. Without detailed teaching and explanations from the master, the student will only learn a lot of forms and flowery techniques. Therefore, many students practice martial arts for many years, but are not able to get the essence of their style. All they have learned are forms. It does not matter how beautiful the forms are: martial art forms without practical usage are called Flower Fist and Brocade Leg (Hua Quan Xiu Tui, 花拳繡腿), which means "useless." Many people I have met said to me that their Gongfu style does not have Shuai Jiao techniques. I asked them to demonstrate their forms and then showed them the Shuai Jiao techniques in the form they just performed. They were very surprised to see Shuai Jiao techniques. Even a simple form like 24 postures Taijiquan has many Shuai Jiao techniques.

Kuai Jiao (快跤), simply means "fast wrestling" in Chinese. During fighting, you will want to find an opportunity to throw down an opponent very quickly and skillfully. The fight should end quickly and you should not be tangled-up with your opponent like a bull fight.

The foundation and principles of Kuai Jiao are based on traditional Chinese wrestling (If the reader is interested in this ancient throwing art, please refer to the Traditional Chinese Wrestling book by Master Liang, Shou-Yu & Tai D. Ngo, coming soon from YMAA Publication Center). In general, most of the Kuai Jiao techniques introduced in this book are based upon traditional Chinese wrestling. This book will introduce about 75 Kuai Jiao techniques for San Shou fighting, and the Traditional Chinese Wrestling book will have more than 300 techniques. If you have a strong foundation in traditional wrestling, it will help your Kuai Jiao skill greatly.

The contents of this book are built upon the foundation of the traditional Chinese Wrestling training. Therefore this book can be used as a reference for martial artists of all different styles. Mastering the techniques in this book will help to bring your fighting ability to a higher level. However, the primary goal of this book is not just for martial artists who love to fight, but rather for all martial arts lovers with an interest in learning and exploring this art. You can easily incorporate these Kuai Jiao techniques into your training. The movements of these techniques are simple and very easy to learn.

The primary goal of this book is to introduce San Shou Kuai Jiao (Fast Wrestling for Free Fighting, 散手快跤) for self defense. However, we will also introduce some ground fighting techniques in the last chapter of this book. One of the reasons is that quite often when you fight, you may fall or be taken to the ground by your opponent. These ground fighting techniques are very useful and also easy to learn.

When practicing, it is not enough to just run through the forms and techniques. You must have a strong basic foundation in order to become good and efficient in the art. This book also introduces some valuable traditional basic training methods with bare hands and with equipment to cultivate and enhance body conditioning and train this art's specialized skills. These methods have passed down from generation to generation. The training methods are simple and refined, and can be fun, challenging and exciting. I hope the reader will enjoy the book and find it helpful.

Here I would like to take this opportunity to express my special thanks to my brother Dr. Yang, Jwing Ming for his encouragement and his many forms of assistance for this and other books.

I would like to thank Al Arsenault for his contribution of all the techniques in the last chapter of this book, which he both demonstrated and wrote. He has studied martial arts since 1971, with special interest in street-applicable techniques from a wide variety of martial arts including Judo, Jujitsu and Qin Na. Mr. Arsenault also trained Shuai Jiao in China. He attained the rank of 3rd degree black belt in Nisei Karate-do in 1986 and is currently founding president of the International Sansho Do Association and is a 4th degree black belt in this discipline. Mr. Arsenault's profession is a Tactical Trainer, Crowd Control Member, Non-Firearms Weapon Expert and First Class Career Constable (since 1979) for the Vancouver Police Department in Canada.

Also I would like to thank my students Sam Masich and Huen Siu Hung for their time and energy and participation in the photo shoots. Sam Masich has studied martial arts since he was young, including Judo and different Chinese internal arts. Sam was member of Canada's first National Wushu Team in 1985. He won two United States National Tai Chi

Championships in 1987 and 1988. He also has a very deep understanding of, and experience in the art of Tai Chi pushing hands and teaches seminars in Canada and the United States.

Huen Siu Hung was also member of Canada's first National Wushu Team in 1985. He has studied a wide variety of Chinese martial arts and has trained in Chinese wrestling since 1985. He has won many gold medals in martial arts competitions in China and the United States.

This book is a collaboration between myself and Mr. Tai D. Ngo. It has been a great pleasure to work with him on this book. He is originally from Viet Nam and his profession is in the field of computers. He loves martial arts and trains very hard. He has participated in many martial arts competitions in the United States, Taiwan, and mainland China, and is the 1992 and 1994 United States National Chinese Martial Arts Competition Grand Champion in men's internal styles.

In addition, I would like to thank Tim Comrie for his photography, Al Loriaux for his help in the last chapter of this book and many YMAA members for general help, including Andrew Murray for his editing.

Liang, Shou-Yu

PREFACE

Mr. Tai D. Ngo

Since I was a boy, learning Gongfu is something that I always wanted to do. I was first introduced to Gongfu by a close friend of my brother's when I was nine years old back in Viet Nam. My training, which only lasted a year, was interrupted by war. During my adolescent years, I traveled and lived in different places in Viet Nam, China and Hong Kong. There were times that martial skills were highly valued for self-protection. Naturally, my desire to learn martial arts was strong, and has not lessened.

It was not until 1985, when I attended Northeastern University in Boston to study Electrical Engineering, that I had the opportunity to meet my teacher Dr. Yang, Jwing-Ming. The introduction was brief and quite unique. I asked Dr. Yang what style of Gongfu he taught. He told me that he taught Shaolin Long Fist, Southern Shaolin White Crane, and Yang Style Taiji. He started to explain and demonstrate a few Qin Na techniques on me. His execution of the Qin Na techniques was most impressive and painful. I dropped immediately to the floor. When I got up, I told him I would be back tomorrow to join the class. I've been training with him ever since.

In the late 80's I had the good fortune to meet Master Liang, Shou-Yu at one of his seminars. His knowledge of internal and external Gongfu styles and of Qigong is vast. Born into a martial arts family, Master Liang had the opportunity to meet many legendary grandmasters. Over the years, I had the opportunity to learn Xingyiquan (Hsing Yi Chuan), Baguazhang, and Chen Style Taijiquan from Master Liang. Also in one of these seminars, I was first introduced to Shan Shou Kuai Jiao. I was immediately fascinated with the effectiveness of the art and started to realize how important Shan Shou Kuai Jiao was to my martial arts training.

Although Master Liang is well known in many styles of Chinese martial arts in China and in North America, few people know that he is an expert in Chinese wrestling. In fact, during his adolescent years, Master Liang won many wrestling matches in private challenges and public competitions. During the political turmoil of the Cultural Revolution in China (1966-1976), Master Liang trained many farmer-students in Wushu and wrestling to defend their homes and villages.

The material in this book is a culmination of Master Liang's many years of extensive experience. I was responsible to help Master Liang translate, compile and write some basic theoretical information. But because of my inexperience in writing martial arts books, all my writing has been checked and corrected by Master Liang and my teacher Dr. Yang, Jwing-Ming.

When my teacher asked me if I could help Master Liang write this book, I hesitated because I knew it would be an important commitment, and also because of my limited understanding of the art. But with the encouragement of Master Liang and Dr. Yang, I gladly accepted the task. It is a great honor to help Master Liang introduce this exciting art to the public.

This book is the first book written in English to introduce the art of Shan Shou Kuai Jiao with complete traditional training methods. For those readers new to the art of Shan Shou Kuai Jiao, this book may serve as a thorough introduction to the art. In chapter 1, we will discuss the basic principles, basic requirements and training stages of the art. In chapter 2 and 3, we will introduce barehand and equipment training for body conditioning. In chapters 4, 5, 6, and 7, we will introduce different varieties of throwing methods. In chapter 8, we will introduce some basic ground control techniques.

Here I would like to take the opportunity to express my gratitude to Master Liang, who believed in me and gave me the honor of helping him write this book, from which I have benefited the most by learning so much. Also, I would like to give special thanks to my teacher Dr. Yang, Jwing-Ming for his encouragement, insight, and technical advice. Thanks to Al Arsenault for sharing his knowledge of ground fighting in chapter 8. Finally, thanks to Andrew Murray for helping to clarify my writing and for general editing.

Tai D. Ngo

Chinese Fast Wrestling for Fighting
The Art of San Shou Kuai Jiao

Chapter 1
General Introduction

一般介紹

1-1. Introduction

San Shou Kuai Jiao (散手快跤) refers to the techniques used in free fighting to take down or throw an opponent. Because *San Shou Kuai Jiao* emphasizes speed, it is known as Fast Wrestling. The words *San Shou* (散手) in Chinese mean free fighting, and imply the use of bare handed martial skills. *Kuai Jiao* (快跤) means quickly downing or throwing an opponent.

Traditionally, Chinese martial arts fighting techniques are divided into four general fighting categories: Ti (踢), Da (打), Shuai (摔), Na (拿). Ti is kicking; Da is striking; Shuai (short for Shuai Jiao, 摔跤) is wrestling; Na is Qin Na (擒拿), i.e. seizing and controlling an opponent's joints and cavities. Generally speaking, when you encounter an opponent in a fight, leg techniques are used in long ranges and hand techniques are used for short ranges.

To become a well-rounded martial artist, you must be proficient in the four basic fighting skills mentioned above. In the past, San Shou competition was held on the Lei Tai (擂臺), a 24 x 24 foot platform 5 feet high. Victory was decided when an opponent was thrown off the Lei Tai or knocked to the floor. Therefore, Shuai Jiao is an important part of San Shou fighting. A martial artist without any Shuai Jiao skills would not easily survive a San Shou match.

Shuai Jiao is believed to be the oldest martial art in China. Its history can be traced back thousands of years. Legend tells that Shuai Jiao already existed during the reign of the Yellow Emperor (Huang Ti, 黄帝 2697 B.C.) and was used to train soldiers. Throughout Chinese history the art has been adopted by governments of different dynasties as a military training method. However, Shuai Jiao was not only used as a tool for military training, but also widely practiced among civilians. It was the civilians who perfected and popularized the art.

In the Song dynasty (960-1278 A.D.), Shuai Jiao skill had reached a very high level and fast wrestling (Kuai Jiao, 快跤) already existed and was very popular. During this period, throws became more complex, and speed and skillfulness of movement was emphasized.

Technically speaking, the foundation and basic principles of San Shou Kuai Jiao are based on traditional Chinese wrestling (Chuan Tong Shuai Jiao, 傳統摔跤) and adapted for combat training. San Shou Kuai Jiao techniques and principles are very simple, effective and—most importantly—quick. Because of its speed and effectiveness, an opponent often does not have a chance to fight back. San Shou Kuai Jiao is an art that does not rely just on muscular strength—it must be done skillfully. It always emphasizes avoiding direct impact with an enemy's power. It also emphasizes getting close to an enemy quickly and using the enemy's power against himself. Because of its effectiveness, San Shou Kuai Jiao has been trained along with all styles of Chinese martial arts for thousands of years.

San Shou Kuai Jiao can cause tremendous physical damage to an opponent. The severity of the damage is dependent on the degree of power used in the technique. Moderate use of power can quickly throw down an opponent and disable his fighting ability. Excessive use of power can permanently injure an opponent. Therefore, the value of San Shou Kuai Jiao has been recognized by Chinese martial artists for centuries. Even with today's modern military technology, San Shou Kuai Jiao is still an important combat skill. In China today it is used to train the police, the military, and special forces.

Differences Between San Shou Kuai Jiao and Other Styles of Wrestling

In general when fighting, the conflict becomes a competition of power, speed, technique, and adaptability to changing situations. The goal is to quickly disable your opponent's fighting ability so that he cannot fight back. When fighting on the street, you cannot risk tangling with your opponent too long. You need to end the fight as soon as possible, especially if you are facing more than one opponent. San Shou Kuai Jiao is perfectly suitable for self-defense on the street because it specializes in throwing techniques to disable an opponent's fighting ability. Throwing techniques can be used whether you initiate the attack or are defending against one. Almost every part of your body can be used against an opponent. The most common body parts used are: head, hands, elbow, shoulder, foot, knees and hips.

As mentioned earlier, San Shou Kuai Jiao is a special kind of martial art technique used to throw or take down an opponent very fast. This art shares many similarities with other wrestling styles, especially traditional Chinese wrestling and Japanese Jujitsu and Judo. This is no surprise because San Shou Kuai Jiao's foundation is based on traditional Chinese wrestling, and traditional Chinese wrestling influenced Jujitsu and Judo.

Many martial arts historians believe that it was Chinese wrestling that greatly influenced the soft arts of Japan. During the late Ming dynasty, a government officer and martial artist named Chen, Yuan-Yun (陳元贇, 1587-1671 A.D. Ming dynasty) fled China to Japan in the year 1659 and later taught martial arts there. This is recorded in Japan's history documents *Collection of Ancestor's Conversations* (先哲叢談), *Volume 2, Biography of Chen, Yuan-Yun* (卷二‧陳元贇傳). The Japanese built a monument to honor his contributions to Japan's martial arts. This monument still stands outside of a temple in Tokyo.

Generally speaking, most San Shou Kuai Jiao techniques were derived from traditional Chinese Wrestling (Shuai Jiao), and Shuai Jiao is the oldest form of Chinese martial arts. However, because Shuai Jiao already existed for thousand of years, it became a complete system by itself. Therefore, Shuai Jiao provides many important foundations for San Shou Kuai Jiao's techniques and development.

Although San Shou Kuai Jiao shares some similarities with traditional wrestling and other arts, from a technical point of view, San Shou Kuai Jiao's technique construction, basic principles, applications and purposes are quite different from the rest. These differences are San Shou Kuai Jiao's distinctive characteristics. In general, we can summarize these differences as follows:

First, compared to traditional Chinese wrestling, Jujitsu and Judo, **San Shou Kuai Jiao emphasizes more speed when throwing.** In contrast, traditional wrestling, Jujitsu and Judo emphasize obtaining good grappling position on an opponent's body or uniform first, and then applying the throw. In this way, it takes more time to throw down an opponent.

Second, **San Shou Kuai Jiao incorporates kicking and punching techniques.** San Shou Kuai Jiao always combines hand and leg techniques. However, traditional wrestling, Jujitsu and Judo, especially the sport varieties, do not emphasize these techniques.

Third, unlike Greco-Roman and free-style wrestling, Jujitsu, and Judo, San Shou Kuai Jiao generally **avoids falling to the ground and grappling too long with an opponent**. One simple reason is that it is dangerous to tangle with an opponent on the ground in a real fight, especially if you face multiple opponents.

These differences do not imply that one style is superior to another. Fighting is a very complicated subject. There are many factors behind victory. Winning a fight depends on situation, timing, location, skills, strength, and the spirit of the individual. It does not depend on the style itself. As a martial artist, keep an open mind to accept and absorb the effective elements of other styles. In turn, it will help to bring your skill to a higher level.

1-2. General Principles of San Shou Kuai Jiao

Like many other different martial art styles, successful strategies for attack and defense will generally follow the style's basic principles and rules. Without understanding the style's principles and rules, you will not achieve a high level of skill. One of the basic principles of San Shou Kuai Jiao is **taking advantage of your opponent's body posture and applying the appropriate techniques at the right time to make your opponent fall.** When applying a San Shou Kuai Jiao technique, you must follow your opponent's body postures and techniques, and know how to borrow your opponent's power and use it against him. For example; when your opponent's body is extend forward, you should not try to throw him backward, and vice versa.

There are two basic elements in a successful throw. **First, the opportunity to quickly throw your opponent depends primarily upon his body posture. Second, you must use the right San Shou Kuai Jiao technique at the right time.** The throw will not be successful if you miss either of the two elements mentioned above.

San Shou Kuai Jiao techniques are concealed by or mixed with hand and leg techniques. The techniques can be defensive or offensive. When used defensively, you must lure an opponent to come in and attack first, or intercept your opponent's attack at the right moment, then apply the appropriate technique. When used offensively, you need to be able to create throwing opportunities by attacking first. Kicks, punches, and fakes will force an opponent to concentrate on defense while you look for the right opportunity to throw him.

Opportunity is an important factor in a fight. But in order to take advantage of an opportunity, timing and decision are important. You need to know how to capitalize on the opportunity when it comes. During fighting, you and your opponent will move and change fighting strategies constantly. Therefore, body postures also change all the time to adjust to new situations. The change in body posture will happen in the blink of an eye. However, there is always a chance that the opponent will make a mistake. When he does, you need to make a quick decision and apply the appropriate technique. If your timing is off or you are indecisive, the opportunity will disappear. And if you pursue a disappearing chance, not only will your efforts be in vain, you may also put yourself in a dangerous position.

In order to be proficient in the art of San Shou Kuai Jiao, not only must you understand the basic principles, but you also need to have many other skills. You need to have the right mindset when facing an opponent; your techniques must be alive, fast and powerful; and you need know how and when to capitalize on opportunities and apply techniques in an ingenious way. Of course, the use of strategy in a fight cannot be ignored.

The following key points are emphasized in San Shou Kuai Jiao training. Each point will be discussed in detail.

1). Coordination of the External and Internal.

2). Grasp the Advantageous Opportunity in a Fight.

3). Techniques Must be Skillful.

4). The Execution of the Techniques Must be Quick.

5). Prepare Mentally.

6). Adapt Strategy Wisely.

1). Coordination of the External and Internal

All proficient Chinese martial artists train the coordination of external physical action (Yang, 陽) and internal mental strength and energy (Yin, 陰). Through this coordination, the entire body is able to manifest power and execute techniques with maximum strength and efficiency. Therefore, external emphasis is on: **hands** (Shou, 手), **eyes** (Yan, 眼), **body** (Shen, 身), **techniques** (Fa, 法), and **stepping** (Bu, 步) and internal emphasis is on: **essence** (Jing, 精), **spirit** (Shen, 神), **internal energy** (Qi, 氣), **muscular strength** (Li, 力), and **Gongfu** or **Kung Fu** (Gong — time and energy, 功). These ten requirements can be considered the root and foundation of Chinese martial arts practice. When these internal and external elements are united and harmonized, the martial techniques will be alive, fast, and powerful. Naturally, since San Shou Kuai Jiao is a part of Chinese martial arts, these ten requirements are also heavily emphasized and practiced in San Shou Kuai Jiao training. If fact, the effectiveness of San Shou Kuai Jiao techniques depends totally on all ten training requirements.

Externally, your eyes must always be on your target. It is the eyes which first observe and detect an opponent's movement, and then a decision is made by the brain. Once a decision is made, the techniques are executed through the hands and the legs, in coordination with the body. That is why it is said: "The eyes arrive, the hands immediately arrive, and the body and stepping also arrive." (Yan Dao Shou Dao, Shen Bu Ye Dao) (眼到，手到，身步也到).

Internally, in order to manifest the external techniques effectively, efficiently, and powerfully, you must learn how to conserve your essence and cultivate and raise your spirit. Then, you can build up abundant Qi (internal energy). When this abundant Qi is directed to the muscles, they manifest strength and power. In addition, once your mind is in a highly alert state, your movements of hands, eyes, body and foot stepping will become agile and will move as one unit. In order to reach this goal of energy manifestation, you must know methods of internal cultivation and how to apply them externally. Without knowing the methods of the training, all of the techniques will be without strong internal support. Consequently, the techniques will be ineffective and weak. Next, let us discuss these ten requirements one by one, beginning with the external.

EXTERNAL:

■ *Hand Drills(Shou Fa, 手法)*

Shou Fa generally refers to the hand techniques used for attack and defense in martial arts. Different martial styles have their own hand techniques and unique ways to manifest the characteristics of the styles. Naturally, San Shou Kuai Jiao also has many different hand techniques and their usage and application depend on the situation. Common hand techniques used in San Shou Kuai Jiao are: grabbing, pulling, thrusting, blocking, holding, lifting, twisting, and pressing. Most importantly, since hands are the main tools in a fight, in order to execute techniques effectively and powerfully, you must train until your hands are strong and fast. In San Shou Kuai Jiao, in order to execute your defensive and offensive techniques effectively, you must be able to extend and withdraw your hands very fast, and grab strongly and tightly. Hand/arm conditioning training will be introduced in chapter 3.

■ *Eye Training (Yan Fa, 眼法)*

A pair of clear and sharp eyes will bring your fighting skills to a higher level. In a fight, the eyes make the first contact and observe your opponent's movement and intention, and then the mind makes judgments to adapt to the situation. Having good vision helps to detect every movement of your opponent and reveals mistakes an opponent makes so you can choose the right decision for an offensive or defensive move. In addition, a good stare can put a lot of mental and psychological pressure on your opponent.

When fighting, look into your opponent's eyes to detect his motivation. When your opponent is scared, you can see that his eyes are not focused but scattered. If he is careless and rude, he will stare back at you. If your opponent is the cunning type, his glance will be subtle. Different fighters have different personalities and different levels of skills; therefore, each will have a very different expression in his eyes.

There are a few ways that you can detect your opponent's intention when you watch his body movements, his facial expressions, and his eyes. When an opponent stares to your left, be wary of an attack to your left side. When an opponent looks down, watch out for his legs. When an opponent attacks with his mouth open, more than likely he will not have much power in his punch or kick. When an opponent attacks with his mouth closed, the power will be strong. Observing shoulder movements is also very important. When the opponent's left shoulder is sinking, very likely he will kick with his right leg. When the opponent's right shoulder moves backward, very likely he will strike with his left hand. Although it will be more complicated in a real fight, body movements generally follow a predictable pattern.

An experienced fighter always watches and uses body movements and eye and facial expressions as a fighting strategy to confuse his opponent, force him to make a wrong decision, and then take advantage of the mistake. In general, eye training is much harder to master than physical techniques and other skills, but it is an invaluable element of martial success.

■ Body Movements (Shen Fa, 身法)

Shen Fa generally refers to the body movement which governs the action of a technique. In order to manifest strong power in the technique executed, you must know how to use your spine and chest to generate the power. The spine and the chest (i.e., torso) are considered to be two big bows which generate power, while the waist acts like a steering wheel which directs the power to the four limbs.

The movements of the torso are divided into four different categories: 1). Changing the chest's direction. 2). Bending and extending the torso forward or backward. 3). Waist rotation and twisting. 4). Using the torso for attacking and defending.

Because all four limbs and the head connect to the body (torso), the movement of the body can lead or control the movement of the head and limbs. The turning and twisting of the body can cause the arms to strike horizontally. When the body is extending forward or withdrawing backward, you can increase the distance for striking or avoiding an opponent's attack. From a power manifestation point of view, the opening and closing of the chest or turning and twisting of the waist helps to store or emit Jin (power).

Besides assisting the movement of the four limbs, the torso can be used for attack and defense. For example, you can use your back or shoulder to press and strike an opponent, or turn and twist the torso to evade an opponent's attack.

Body movements in the martial arts should be lively and should emphasize the use of the waist. Also, body movements must be quick. Even if your limbs are fast, if your body does not have speed, the techniques will not be fast and effective. Therefore, the body is the foundation of the hands and legs. The hands and legs can move fast only when the body can move fast. You should always avoid bodily stiffness. A relaxed body is the key to agility and swiftness.

■ Strategy and Techniques (Fa/Ji Fa, 技法)

Fa means the method or technique. In a martial context, it means fighting techniques and strategies. Good fighting techniques act as a channel for speed and power, to direct the speed and power efficiently and effectively. If you have speed and power but no techniques, you will be a less effective fighter. Conversely, if you know many techniques but lack speed and power, your techniques will be of little use.

Good techniques must be learned from experienced masters. A master is just like a coach in sports—without a good experienced coach, even if you have good players, your team may not win.

When you learn techniques from a master, you will also learn the fighting strategies. Generally, fighting strategies are obtained from experience. The more experience a master has, the more he knows how to handle different situations. Not only that, he will know how to set up an opponent and create opportunities to make every technique effective, efficient, and powerful.

■ *Stepping (Bu Fa, 步法)*

Bu Fa generally refers to the stepping techniques or footwork used to move and change direction. Bu Fa has the purpose of moving the body forward and backward, dodging left and right, and increasing the ability to extend, twist, and turn the body. Foot stability is the foundation of balanced movement. The quickness of the footwork will increase the technique's speed and power. Skillful stepping is the foundation of agility.

Chinese martial arts demonstrate a variety of Bu Fa. Aside from common stepping methods, many styles have unique footwork that reflects the principles behind those styles. For example: Taijiquan's (太極拳) Taiji Bu (Taiji Stepping, 太極步); Baguazhang's (八卦掌) Tang Ni Bu (Muddy Stepping, 蹚泥步); Xingyiquan's (形意拳) Cun Bu (Inch stepping, 寸步), Ji Bu (Urgent stepping, 疾步), and Zuan Bu (Drill stepping, 躦步), etc.

In a fight, your footwork is constantly changing to adjust to the situation. Proper positioning and speed can put you in the most advantageous position to execute your techniques. When you can move fast and occupy the most advantageous position, you will put your opponent in an urgent, defensive position. The common stepping techniques used in San Shou Kuai Jiao will be introduced in chapter 2.

Next we will examine the internal elements in the Coordination of External and Internal.

INTERNAL:

■ *Essence (Jing, 精)*

Jing means essence, the most refined organic material in your body, which you inherited from your parents. In fact, it is the Jing which decides how strong and healthy you will be. Chinese medicine believes human Jing is stored in the kidneys. When the Jing is abundant and of good quality, you will have a strong physical body, abundant Qi, and a high spirit. Therefore, learning how to conserve your essence has been an important part of Chinese martial arts training. There are a few things that may affect the storage of your essence.

1. Too much sex. This applies to males. According to Chinese medicine, when a man engages in too much sexual activity, his kidneys will be overworked and the production of the essence to supply the body's needs will be significantly reduced. Therefore, a martial artist must learn to regulate his sex life. It has also been discovered in Chinese martial arts society that if a man has sex before combat, his energy and endurance will be low and he can easily be defeated.

2. Too much training without rest. A smart martial artist will know how to train hard but also know how to relax and allow his body to recover. When a body is over-exercised, the kidneys and liver will be too Yang, or too positive, which can result in physical and mental fatigue. When this happens, you will not be able to keep your mental center in the fight. Consequently, your spirit will be low and your judgment poor.

3. Unhealthy lifestyle. Another way to damage the storage and the manifestation of the essence is a poor lifestyle—excessive drinking, smoking, a lack of sleep, and poor eating habits. When this happens, both the physical and spiritual body will be affected, and your Qi will also be weak and deficient.

Therefore, in order to perform your martial skill effectively and efficiently, the first thing you should concern yourself with is how to preserve and protect your essence. Essence (Jing, 精), Spirit (Shen, 神), and Internal Energy (Qi, 氣) are considered the three treasures (San Bao, 三寶) in Chinese Qigong and martial arts society.

■ *Spirit (Shen, 神)*

Shen is spirit, or morale. When your spirit is high, your fighting techniques can be executed skillfully and powerfully. In Chinese Qigong society, it is believed that it is the essence stored in the body which makes the production of Qi strong (Lian Jing Hua Qi, 練精化氣). When the Qi is abundant and circulating strongly, the Qi can be led to the brain to raise the spirit, which can strengthen your will and motivation.

It is because of this reason that Jing-Shen (Essence-Spirit) is commonly used together and referred to as the "spirit of vitality." It also reflects the energy (Qi) level of your body. When your spirit is high the Qi can be directed efficiently to energize the physical body to its maximum.

Learning how to raise your spirit of vitality is an important part of Chinese martial arts training. When your spirit is high, you will be brave and confident. It is said: "Yi Dan, Er Li, San Gongfu" (一膽, 二力, 三功夫). This means: "First, bravery; second, power; and third, technique." From this, you can see bravery, generated by a high spirit (fighting morale), is the most important element for a martial artist to have.

To conclude, when your spirit is high it will reflect externally in your face and eyes, which shows your opponent your confidence and bravery. Therefore, when you encounter an opponent, you must first raise your spirit yet remain calm. Physically, when your spirit is high your Qi is abundant and able to energize the muscles and tendons to their maximum efficiency. When this happens, your body will become more agile, speedy, and powerful.

■ *Internal Energy (Qi, 氣)*

As mentioned earlier, Qi is one of the three treasures for maintaining your life force. Qi generally refers to universal energy, and also to the energy circulating in human and animal bodies. To Chinese martial artists, Qi is the root and foundation of physical strength. Through correct breathing training and mental concentration, Qi can be built up to a stronger and more abundant level in the Lower Dan Tian (Xia Dan Tian, 下丹田). When this internal energy is sent to the external physical body, it becomes martial power (Jin) and significantly improves the effectiveness of the techniques you execute.

When you encounter an opponent, you must keep your mind calm and breathe naturally. Use reverse breathing to sink your Qi to the Lower Dan Tian to prevent your body and mind from getting too excited, which can result in shallow breathing. When you are excited and breathe shallowly, your Qi will rise upward and become weak. In this case, your root will also be shallow, making it easier for your opponent to throw you down.

In addition, when you are excited and breathing fast, you will become fatigued and lose your endurance. In order to maintain your endurance and keep your fighting spirit high, you must learn how to use and control your Qi efficiently. When this internal energy is manipulated properly, it will maximize your physical strength. To learn more about Qi and Qigong, especially for martial purposes, refer to the book *The Essence of Shaolin White Crane,* by Dr. Yang, Jwing-Ming.

■ *Power/Strength (Li, 力)*

The general understanding of Li is muscular power (force) generated by the physical body. It also implies the martial power (Jin, 勁) of martial arts training. Jin is generally defined as **martial power in which your physical body is energized by Qi and the spirit to its maximum efficiency and potential.** All Chinese martial arts styles train Jin. Although there are many different ways of Jin training in Chinese martial arts, its theory and principles remain the same.

In order to make the San Shou Kuai Jiao techniques effective and powerful, you must also train Jin. There are many different kinds of San Shou Kuai Jiao Jin training. For example: Inch Jin (Cun Jin, 寸勁), Explosive Jin (Bao Fa Jin, 爆發勁), Extend/Stretch Jin (Beng Jin, 弸勁), Ingenuity Jin (Qiao Jin, 巧勁), Penetrate/ Thrusting Jin (Tong Jing, 捅勁), Twisting Jin (Ning Jin, 撸勁), etc. When Jin is properly applied to a technique, the technique becomes more powerful and alive.

A proficient martial artist should always avoid using Jin directly against an opponent's Jin. You should be able to manifest Jin naturally, and either as hard or as soft as necessary. When the Jin is too hard, the power will not be alive and smooth and can be easily neutralized by your opponent. If it is too soft, then the power will not be strong enough to execute the technique effectively and powerfully. Some Jin training methods will be introduced in chapter 2 and chapter 3 of this book. For more information on Jin training, refer to the book *Tai Chi Theory & Martial Power,* by Dr. Yang, Jwing-Ming.

■ *Gongfu/Kung Fu (Gong, 功)*

Gong generally refers to the level of martial skill attained by the martial artist. It includes body conditioning, internal mind and Qi cultivation, martial techniques, and power. In some styles, Gong often refers to special skill levels which take a great effort of energy and time to train. Therefore, Gong has been commonly used to measure the level of effectiveness and strength of the power in martial techniques.

Gongfu/Kung Fu (功夫) literally means "energy-time." It also refers to any study, learning, or practice which requires patience, energy, and time to learn or accomplish. Since practicing Chinese martial arts requires a great deal of time and energy, Chinese martial arts are also commonly called Gongfu.

To become a proficient San Shou Kuai Jiao expert, your San Shou Kuai Jiao Gongfu level must be excellent in all areas—technique, speed, power, spirit, etc. When your opponent is fast, you must be faster. When your opponent is powerful, you should be stronger, fiercer, and more skillful. Your endurance should be superior. In all, your Gongfu (basic body and mental conditioning and skills) has to be of the highest level in order to win. Keep practicing basic skills diligently and you will make your San Shou Kuai Jiao Gongfu more proficient.

2). Opportunity (Shi Ji, 時機)

In a fight, you must be able to seize the opportunity when it comes. Opportunity can be found or created. It is based upon your opponent's body gestures, techniques, or mistakes made during the fight. When there is an opportunity, the proper San Shou Kuai Jiao technique must be applied correctly in order to throw your opponent.

Opportunity comes and goes rather quickly. If there is an opportunity and you are not able to catch it, or you hesitate to make a decision, it will vanish in the blink of an eye. Once the opportunity has passed and you still try to apply a technique, you may be giving your opponent a chance to reverse the situation. For example, when your opponent attacks you with a right punch to your face, you may quickly dodge to the right and use your left hand to grab his right wrist to control him, and then apply an appropriate San Shou Kuai Jiao technique to throw him down. But if your timing is wrong and reaction is slow, his arm has already been pulled back before you can grab it. You have missed the chance. If you continue to execute the grab, your opponent can take the opportunity to attack you.

Opportunity can be created. An experienced fighter is able to use strategies and tricks to open his opponent to attack. Of course, it is not easy to catch every possible opportunity during a fight. Your skills and knowledge will grow along with your experience, but not without hard work. Therefore, the more you are able to practice with different partners, the better you will increase this experience, and train yourself to recognize and take advantage of opportunities.

3). Ingenuity (Qiao, 巧)

Ingenuity is the skill in San Shou Kuai Jiao training that teaches you how to apply your techniques cleverly. In fact, ingenuity must be combined with others skills such as reaction, speed, endurance, and durability of the body as a whole. It is the most advanced product of all martial arts skills combined. In a complex situation such as a fight, you can not just rely on one or two particular skills to defeat your opponent. Instead, you must use techniques, footwork, the ability to move your body well, the ability to use strategies, and the ability to improvise and take advantage of situations.

Ingenuity is the ability to take advantage of situations. Each individual person will apply this skill differently. If you are physically stronger than your opponent, take that as your advantage. But if you are not as strong as your opponent, you can not blindly match muscle power against muscle power. You must observe your opponent's movement carefully and then apply appropriate techniques cleverly. In order to improve this type of skill, reaction ability and the use of strategy must be emphasized. Ingenuity will improve through training, analysis, and experience.

4). Speed (Su Du, 速度)

Speed is one of the most important elements in martial arts training. Without proper speed, all the martial arts techniques in the world will not help you. There are different types of speed emphasized in martial arts training. Common speed training emphasizes the quickness of the eyes, hands, body, legs, footwork, and mind.

The most important among them is the speed of mind. The mind is the control center of the body. Although the speed of the entire physical body is important, the mind has the most important role in deciding which reactions to perform and what strategy to apply to the situation. If your mind is uncertain and slow to respond, then your decisions will not be firm and your reactions will be slow. This means that your hands and feet will also be slow, since their movements are controlled by the mind. Mind also plays the main role in directing the eyes to observe and react to your opponent's movements. When the state of your mind is firm and your spirit is high, every part of your body will able to respond to your opponent's strategy. On the other hand, when you lack focus and your spirit is low, your reaction will be slow.

As we mentioned above, the mind controls the speed of the physical body, and the reaction time of the mind plays an important role in the art of fighting. Therefore, reaction must also be emphasized in training. Generally speaking, reaction is the ability of your body to respond to sudden changes. The ability to react fast in San Shou Kuai Jiao is very important. When fighting, you and your opponent's body gestures and techniques change very quickly. To be able to react to sudden changes during a fight, you must not only have appropriate techniques, but also good speed.

Speed is a key factor for a successful throw in San Shou Kuai Jiao. Your hands and legs must coordinate. There is a saying when applying San Shou Kuai Jiao techniques in fight; "Eyes like lighting; Hands like an arrow; Waist like a coiling snake; Legs like a drill" (Yan Si Shan Dian; Shou Si Jian; Yao Si Pan She; Jiao Si Zuan) (眼似閃電，手似箭。腰似盤蛇，腳似鑽。). The above saying points out the importance of the speed of eyes, hands, body and legs which San Shou Kuai Jiao depends on to win the fight. With good speed, your techniques will be more sudden and not give your opponent time to react to your attack. If your movements are agile and lively, your opponent will not be able to discern your intention until it is too late.

The important point is that speed and reaction are a crucial part of San Shou Kuai Jiao training. If you have only good techniques but no speed and reaction, you will not be able to apply the throwing techniques efficiently. Therefore, speed and reaction must be emphasized in San Shou Kuai Jiao training.

5). State Of Mind (Xin Li Juang Tai, 心理狀態)

State of mind is the expression of emotional activities of the brain during a fight. State of mind can be seen through body movement, and also in the eyes and facial expression. State of mind is often referred to as "spirit" in martial arts.

All activities in the body and mind are closely related. Mentality is the main force behind your techniques, speed and power. Of course, your mental and emotional state of mind are dependent on your level of skill. The higher the level of skill you have, the higher your confidence and spirit will be.

A fight is not just a contest of fists. It is also a contest of minds. When facing an opponent, the first thing you must do is raise your spirit and psychologically feel an advantage over your opponent. In fighting, you must have confidence and courage, and believe that you can defeat your opponent. Keep yourself calm and do not hesitate. Dare to fight against your opponent. Such fearless spirit is a requirement that a martial artist must have. Psychologically you have to believe that you are stronger than your opponent and you can overcome any obstacle to defeat him. There is an old saying in Chinese "Liang Qiang Xiang Yu; Yong Zhe Sheng" (兩強相遇，勇者勝) , which means "When two strong (fighters) meet, the brave one will win." Bravery is the state of mind filled with courage and fearlessness.

Another important aspect of the state of mind is mental self-control. The control ability will first appear in the stability of emotion (feeling). When facing a good fighter, you must keep calm and breathe naturally, or use reverse breathing to help prevent getting excited. Keep your facial expression solemn and natural. In this way, you show your opponent nothing. But in return, you put psychological pressure on your opponent. Act bravely or seriously inside (state of mind) and indolent (casually) outside. In a fight, you must control your emotion. Do not rush to attack blindly without understanding your opponent. Your opponent may very well play the same game that you are playing. Observe every detail of the situation. Control yourself mentally and do not get excited in either an advantageous or disadvantageous position.

6). Strategy (Zhan Shu, 戰術)

In order to do well in a fight, not only do you need to have superior spirit, techniques and skills, but you also need to have the ability to apply strategies in a fight. An experienced fighter always knows how to take advantage of the situation and is able to create opportunities by using fakes and confusing or intimidating his opponent.

Faking techniques can be divided into three different kinds. First is the fake that conceals a real technique. Second is the fake used to set a trap by purposely opening yourself to your opponent. The third is used to provoke or enrage an opponent, to make the opponent angry so that he will lose control, and will more likely make careless mistakes that you can take advantage of.

The effectiveness of using fakes in fight depends upon your ability to analyze and compare your own and your opponent's real strengths, the ability to make the fake look real, self control, and the ingenuity to use your advantages against your opponent's shortcomings. However, you should not underestimate your opponent's skill, and never overestimate yourself.

1-3. The Three Training Stages of San Shou Kuai Jiao

The training and development of San Shou Kuai Jiao skills generally goes in three stages. The first stage is learning the basic skills of San Shou Kuai Jiao. The second stage is to master those basic skills. The third stage is to be able to use those skills naturally and creatively in real situations.

1. The Fundamental Stage:

San Shou Kuai Jiao training must start with basic training for body conditioning. Through basic training you improve your speed, power, confidence and body coordination.

In this stage of training, you will practice single San Shou Kuai Jiao techniques until they are smooth and accurate. This stage emphasizes techniques, footwork, body coordination and understanding the application of each technique. Also, solo forms and equipment training will improve endurance and power. Proper development of one technique requires long hard training. Above all, the most important element is the development of your Will, Bravery and Alertness.

2. Mastering and Specializing in Techniques Stage:

According to your own body potential and condition, select the San Shou Kuai Jiao techniques that suit you most. Each individual's body height, weight, shape, strength and condition is different. Therefore, you should choose techniques that suit your own condition and specialize in them. The benefit of selecting favorite techniques is that it boosts enthusiasm and speeds up the learning process and understanding of the techniques.

At this point you should have a very solid foundation of San Shou Kuai Jiao techniques, body conditioning and other important requirements. Also in this stage, you should further explore the concepts of speed and fighting distance to further improve your attacking and defending abilities. Continue to polish your San Shou Kuai Jiao techniques to make them natural, so that your body will react automatically and correctly. At this stage of training, you will start to form your own specialized San Shou Kuai Jiao techniques and fighting strategy.

3. Refining Stage:

With the combination of solid basic skills and specialized skills, this is the time to test the abilities you have acquired and apply them in more competitive environments, like sparring and competitions. At this stage you will hone your basic skills and train your ingenuity and fighting strategies. To reach this level requires a strong will, a commitment to hard work, thoughtful analysis, and the clarity of mind to know your goals and see how best to achieve them.

Chapter 2
Basic Training

基本訓練

2-1. Introduction

Basic training is the root and foundation of San Shou Kuai Jiao. This training teaches the fundamental skills and principles of the art. You need to understand and master the basic skills in order to apply San Shou Kuai Jiao techniques effectively. Also, basic training helps you build a solid foundation for further advancement. An effective San Shou Kuai Jiao technique requires whole-body coordination, including hands, body movement, footwork (stepping), and falling. Basic training develops this coordination, along with good posture and good body control. Furthermore, basic training will help you to improve your strength, speed, endurance and technical accuracy. The training methods introduced in this chapter are essential for proficiency in San Shou Kuai Jiao. You should learn and master these basics before practicing the San Shou Kuai Jiao techniques in later chapters.

In this chapter, we will introduce some warm up exercises, stances, footwork, beginning entering training, and falling techniques.

2-2. Warm Up Exercises

The warm up is an important part of every workout. Warm up will help you to stimulate your joints, muscles, and the central nervous system of your body. Also, warm up exercises will help you improve your flexibility and strengthen muscles and tendons in your body. Your body should be warm and loose before you start your practice. In this section, we will introduce some typical exercises. Practitioners can add their own exercises to fit their personal needs.

1. Waist Rotation 小涮腰

For warming up and loosening the waist muscles.

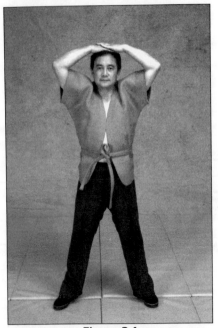

Figure 2-1

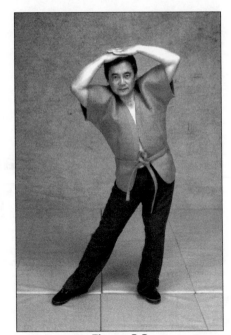

Figure 2-2

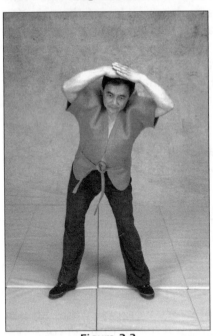

Figure 2-3

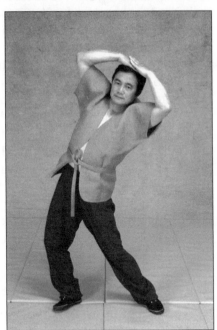

Figure 2-4

Training Method:

Stand with your legs shoulder-width apart and place both hands on top of your head. Rotate your waist clockwise repeatedly and then counterclockwise (Figures 2-1 to 2-5).

2. **Large Waist Rotation** 大涮腰

Increases waist flexibility and muscle strength.

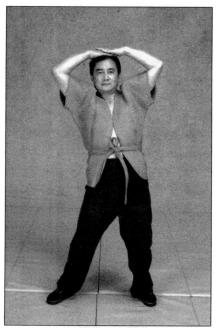

Figure 2-5

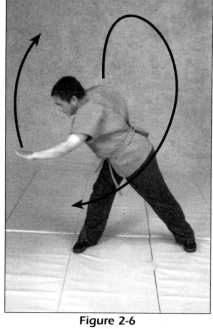

Figure 2-6

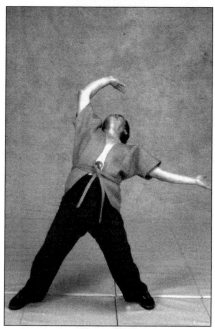

Figure 2-7

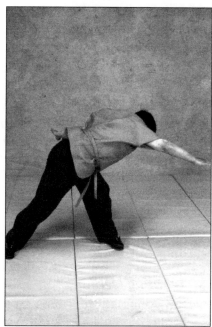

Figure 2-8

Training Method:

Stand with both legs shoulder width apart. Extend both arms to the sides. Bend the torso towards your left leg (Figure 2-6) and make large, sweeping circles from left to right and back to the starting position. Be sure to make complete circles and emphasize moving from the waist. The arms should be loose and extended and the circular motion should be smooth and continuous (Figures 2-7 and 2-8 and 2-9). Repeat this exercise as many times as you want, and then change to the opposite direction.

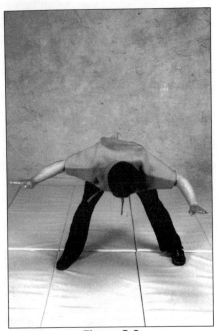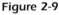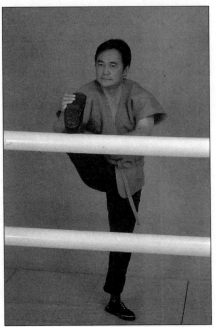

Figure 2-9	Figure 2-10

3. Front Leg Press 正壓腿

Increases the flexibility and strength of the leg muscles and tendons.

Training Method:

Put your right foot on a stretch bar higher than your waist, with your body facing forward. Straighten both the leg on the bar and the leg on the ground. With a straight back, bend forward towards your right foot and try to touch your chest to your leg. (Figure 2-10). Repeat 20 to 30 times and then change legs.

4. Sideways Leg Press 側壓腿

Increases the flexibility and strength of the leg muscles and tendons. Also helps to increase the turning angle of the hip joints.

Training Method:

Put your right foot on a stretch bar higher than your waist. Your torso should face sideways. Keep both legs straight and press your body sideways toward your right. Try to touch your right leg with your right shoulder (Figure 2-11). Repeat 20 to 30 times and then change legs.

5. Backward Leg Press 后壓腿

Increases the flexibility and strength of the back and legs.

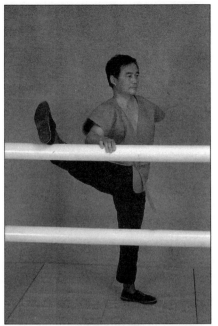

Figure 2-11

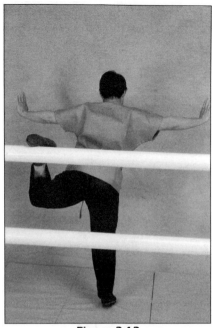

Figure 2-12

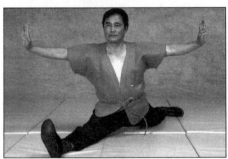

Figure 2-13

Training Method:

Put your left foot on a stretch bar higher than your waist. The knee should be bent and your back should face the bar. Keep your right leg straight, keep your head up and press your body backward (Figure 2-12). Repeat 20 to 30 times and then change legs.

6. Leg Splits 劈叉

Increases the flexibility and strength of the leg muscles and tendons.

Training Method:

Keep both legs straight, one in front and one in back. Use one hand on either side of the body for support. Press downward so that your legs touch the floor. Make sure to keep your hip straight and your torso facing the front leg (Figure 2-13). Repeat 20 to 30 times, and then switch sides. To avoid injury, start slowly and gradually increase both the repetitions and the depth of the split.

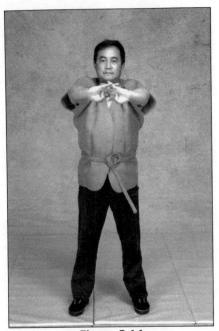

Figure 2-14

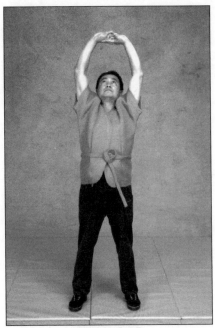

Figure 2-15

7. **Tendon Stretching** 伸筋

Increases the flexibility of the back and legs.

Training Method:

Stand with both legs straight and shoulder-width apart. Lock your fingers together and extend the arms forward at shoulder height. Then raise your hands above your head. From this position, bend forward from the waist until your hands touch the floor. Staying bent, wrap your arms around your calves and pull your head towards your shins. The legs must remain straight at all times. Stay in this position for 10 to 30 seconds and repeat as many times as you like (Figures 2-14 to 2-17).

8. **Diagonal Stretching** 合臥襠

Increases the flexibility and strength of the waist and legs.

Training Method:

Open both legs wider than your shoulders. Keep your torso straight and bend forward from the waist. Try to touch the floor with your forehead while keeping your legs straight. (Figure 2-18). Then move to the right leg and then the left leg. Try to bring your forehead to your foot. Both hands should hold the leg (Figures 2-19 and 2-20).

9. **Front Kick** 正踢腿

Helps to improve flexibility, leg movement, and body stability.

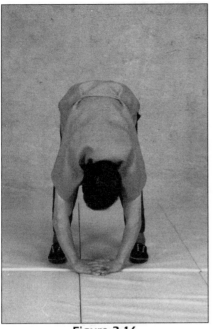

Figure 2-16

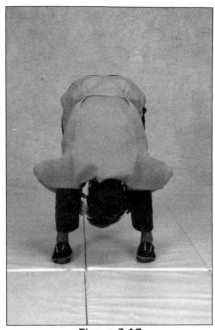

Figure 2-17

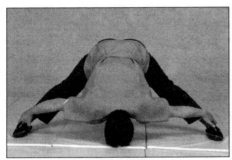

Figure 2-18

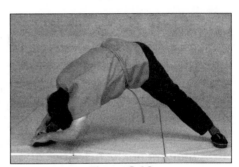

Figure 2-19

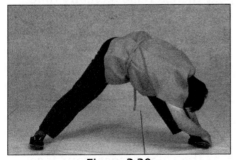

Figure 2-20

Training Method:

Stand with one foot forward, both knees slightly bent, and the heel of the rear foot slightly lifted. Stretch both arms to the sides at shoulder height. Kick upward as high as you can with the rear leg. The kicking leg must keep straight with the toes locked in. Don't bend your back when kicking. The heel of the supporting leg should not leave the ground (Figure 2-21). Repeat the kick as many times as you like and then change sides.

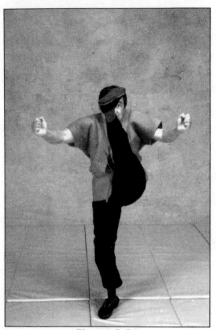

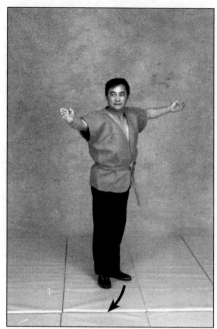

| Figure 2-21 | Figure 2-22 |

10. Side Kick 側踢腿

Helps to improve flexibility, leg movement, and body stability.

Training Method:

Stand sideways and extend both hands out to the sides (Figure 2-22). Cross your left foot in front of your right (Figure 2-23) and then kick with your right leg sideways and up towards your right shoulder. Keep the kicking leg straight and lock in the toes. Simultaneously, bring your right hand down to waist height and your left hand in front and above your head (Figure 2-24). Bring the kicking leg straight down. Repeat the exercise as many time as you like, then change legs.

11. Outside Crescent Kick 擺蓮腿

Increases the flexibility in the hip joints.

Training Method:

Stand with the legs shoulder width apart and extend both hands out to the sides. Turn your body slightly to your left and sweep the right leg upward from the left to the right across your face and downward to your right. Keep your kicking leg straight and lock your toes (Figures 2-25 and 2-26). Remember to use the waist to generate power. Repeat as many times as you like and then switch legs.

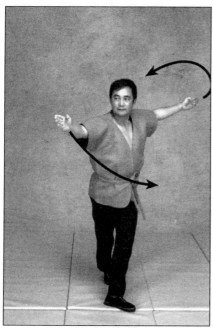

Figure 2-23

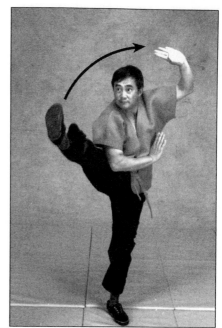

Figure 2-24

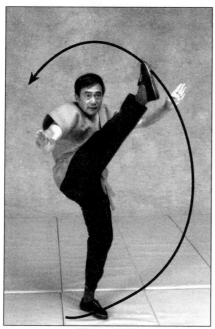

Figure 2-25

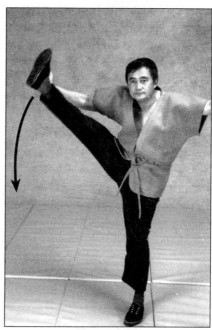

Figure 2-26

12. Inside Crescent Kick 裡合腿

Increases the flexibility in the hip joints.

Training Method:

Stand with the legs shoulder width apart and extend both hands out to the sides. Sweep your right leg upward and out to the right and then across to the left. Keep the kicking leg straight and lock

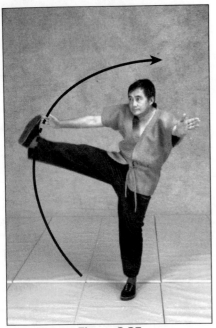

Figure 2-27

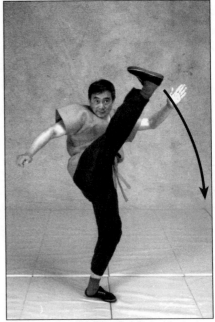

Figure 2-28

in your toes (Figures 2-27 and 2-28). Remember to use the waist to generate power. Repeat as many times as you like and then switch legs.

2-3. San Shou Kuai Jiao Basic Stances and Leg Training 散手快跤基本腿功

Basic stance training and basic leg training are important in San Shou Kuai Jiao. They include fundamental techniques specially designed for San Shou Kuai Jiao. It is very common that basic stances and basic legs techniques are blended together in the training. Stance training will help you develop the correct postures for San Shou Kuai Jiao applications. Basic leg training will help you to improve the mobility of the legs and body movement. Combining stances and leg training is an effective way to gain good body control, strength, balance, and whole-body coordination.

1. Back Hook 跪腿

For leg hooking and supporting leg stability training.

Training Method:

Stand with both legs shoulder width apart, both hands on your waist (Figure 2-29). Hook your right leg upward from behind with the sole of the foot facing up (Figure 2-30). Keep the supporting leg stable and repeat the exercise as many times as you like, and then switch legs.

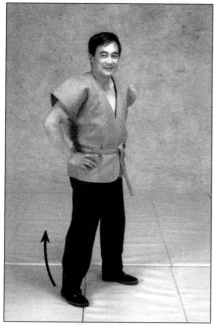

Figure 2-29

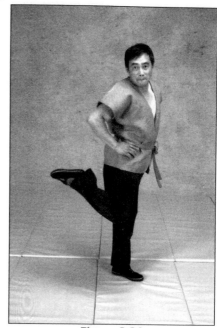

Figure 2-30

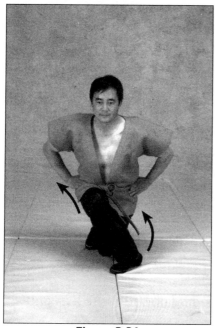

Figure 2-31

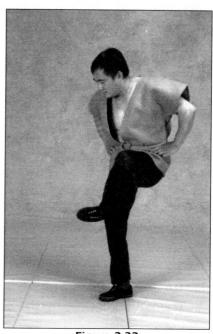

Figure 2-32

2. **Pulling Out the Leg** 抽腿

Increases leg mobility and strength. For example: when your leg is pinched by your opponent, you can easily pull it out for a counterattack.

Training Method:

Sit down with your left leg crossed and on top of your right (Figure 2-31). Stand up and lift your right leg with the knee bent

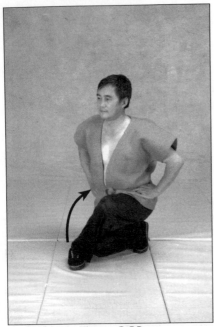

Figure 2-33

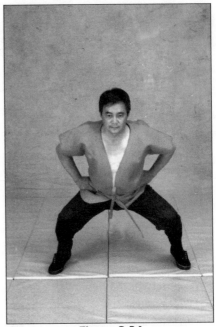

Figure 2-34

(Figure 2-32). Then step to the right. Then lift your left leg in the same manner, cross in front of the right and squat down (Figure 2-33). Switch right and left repeatedly.

3. Squat Down Hook Kicking 蹲踢

For stability training and hooking or kicking an opponent's heel.

Training Method:

Squat down in Horse Stance (Figure 2-34), then kick upwards to your left with the right leg. Pull your toes back, keep the leg straight, and let the kicking leg's heel brush the floor on its way up. Pull both hands from left to right to create symmetry power (Figure 2-35). Keep the supporting leg bent throughout the kick. Alternate with both legs to repeat the exercise.

4. Turning in Bow Stance 大轉腳

Trains the turning, twisting and exploding power of the legs and hips.

Training Method:

Start in Right Bow Stance (Figure 2-36) and turn your body, using both heels, to Left Bow Stance. While you are turning, the right heel pushes into the ground to create the explosive twisting power of the legs and hips. Repeat the exercise by switching from left to right.

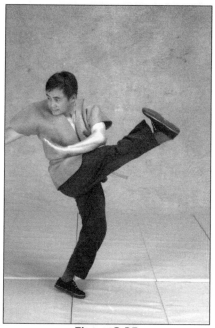

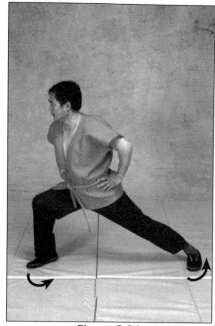

<table>
</table>

Figure 2-35   Figure 2-36

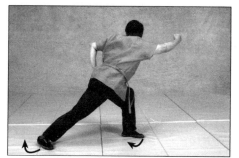
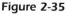

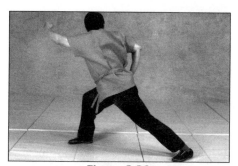

Figure 2-37   Figure 2-38

5. Extending the Body 長腰

Trains the combined power of body turning and extending the power of the body and arms to drag an opponent or break free from an opponent's grab.

Training Method:

Start in Left Bow Stance with the left fist close to the waist. Your right arm extends foward with the right fist closed (Figure 2-37). Turn your body to the right on both heels. While you are turning, the left heel pushes into the ground to create the explosive twisting power. Simultaneously, pull the right hand back to your waist, extend the left hand as far forward as you can and turn your body to the right. Look back all the way to your right (Figure 2-38). Repeat the same exercise in the opposite direction for the left side. Change from side to side as many times as you like.

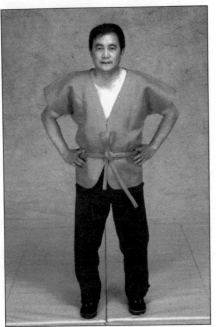

Figure 2-39

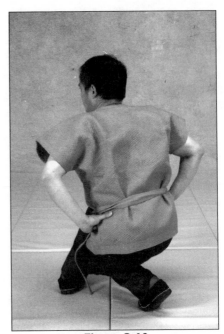

Figure 2-40

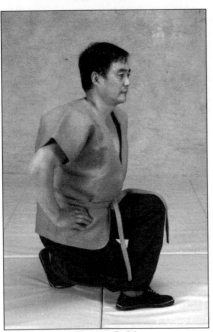

Figure 2-41

6. Sitting and Crossing Leg

少轉腿

For leg flexibility and strength and body balance.

Training Method:

Stand with both legs shoulder width apart (Figure 2-39). Pivot 180 degrees to your right on your right heel and left toes and lower your body so that your right leg will be on top of the left (Figure 2-40). Twist back up to a standing position and repeat the same exercise in the opposite direction (Figure 2-41). Continue to pivot from side to side as many times as you like.

7. Jumping Training 跳八扇

For speed, body mobility, and coordination training.

Training Method:

Stand with feet shoulder width apart (Figure 2-42). Both legs jump up and land in a Left Bow Stance. Simultaneously, twist

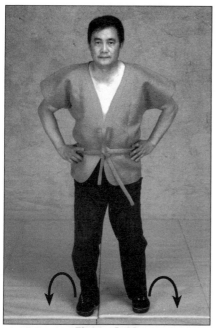

Figure 2-42

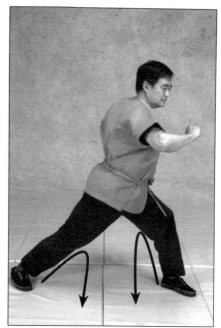

Figure 2-43

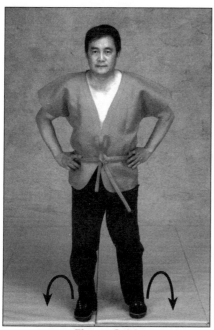

Figure 2-44

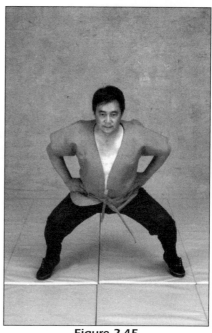

Figure 2-45

your body to your left, pull the left hand back to the waist, and extend the right hand in front of your body (Figure 2-43). Both legs jump up from Left Bow Stance to the original position (Figure 2-44). From the original position, both legs jump up and land in a Horse Stance (Figure 2-45). From Horse Stance you can repeat the exercise for Right Bow Stance.

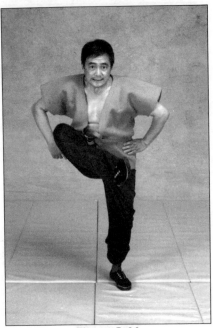

Figure 2-46

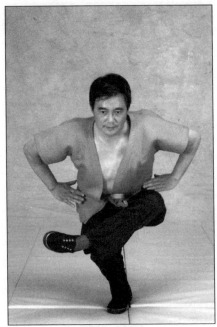

Figure 2-47

8. Coiling Leg 盤腿

Trains you to lift your leg quickly and easily. Usually used to escape low kicks or lower leg controlling techniques. This exercise will also help to loosen up your hip joint.

Training Method:

Stand with both legs shoulder width apart. Shift your body weight to your left leg and lift your right leg upwards at least as high as your knee (Figure 2-46). Put your right leg down and repeat with your left leg. Alternate both legs as many times as you like.

9. Stationary Coiling Leg 盤腿耗椿

For leg and knee strength, balance, and stretching the hip joints.

Training Method:

Put both hands on your waist and squat down. Put your left leg on top of your right knee. Stay in this position for at least 1 to 5 minutes (Figure 2-47). Change to the other leg and repeat the exercise. Keep your back straight and slowly increase the length of time you can hold this position.

10. Coiling Leg and Kicking Backward 盤腿扔空

For leg hooking and blocking techniques.

Training Method:

Start from the stationary coiling leg position with the right leg on

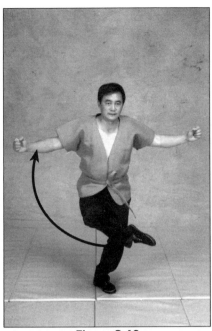

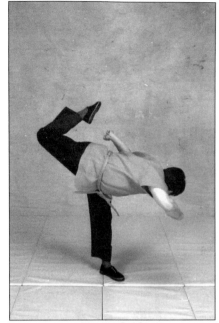

Figure 2-48   Figure 2-49

top and both arms extended to the sides (Figure 2-48). Twist your body to your left on the ball of your left foot, swing your right leg down and backward, then hook the leg up as high as you can, bending the knee and pointing the toe. Simultaneously, pull your left hand back to the waist and the right hand upward then downward to your left so that both arms move in a large circular motion. Bend forward, keep your chin tucked in, and look to your left (Figure 2-49). Change to the other leg and repeat this exercise in the opposite direction. Always keep your supporting leg slightly bent so you will not lose your balance when kicking backward.

2-4. Basic San Shou Kuai Jiao Entering Training 快跤基本步法

In order to apply San Shou Kuai Jiao techniques effectively, you need to have proper footwork (stepping) and stances. All the San Shou Kuai Jiao techniques require certain entering methods to complete the throws. But keep in mind that the entering skill is built on the foundation of the stances and footwork methods already introduced. Footwork allows you to control your body balance and many San Shou Kuai Jiao techniques require proper stepping to complete the throw.

Without a proper way to get close to your opponent, your San Shou Kuai Jiao techniques will not be effective. Thus, entering skills are very important. Although some San Shou Kuai Jiao techniques do not require you to get very close to your opponent to throw him, a smooth and quick entering move will give your opponent no time to react and will put you at an advantage.

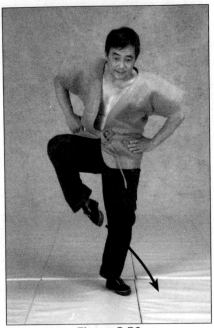
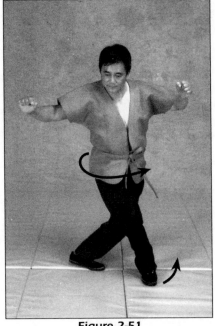

Figure 2-50   Figure 2-51

In this section, we will introduce a few entering methods commonly used in San Shou Kuai Jiao. You can practice them solo or with a partner.

1. Front Cross Step Entering 蓋步入

Training Method:

Stand with your feet shoulder width apart and squat down slightly. Lift your right foot and cross it in front of your left foot (Figures 2-50 and 2-51). Pivot your body to the left on the balls of the feet and thrust your right hip backward. Keep your body posture low (Figure 2-52). Spring up on both of your knees and keep the right hip driving upward, while simultaneously bending forward to your left. Your left hand should pull downward then upward to the back and your right hand should pull downward to your left to trace a large circular motion. Keep your chin tucked in and look back to your left (Figure 2-53). Repeat the exercise as many times as you like and switch to the other side and repeat the movements in the opposite direction.

2. Back Cross Step Entering 背入

Training Method:

This entering technique is almost exactly the same as the previous technique **Front Cross Step Entering** except that from the starting position, the left foot steps behind the right foot. The rest of the movements are the same. Train both sides as many times as you want (Figures 2-54 to 2-56).

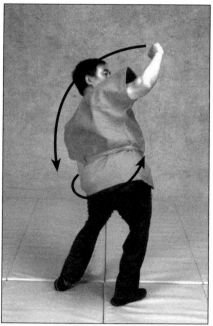

Figure 2-52

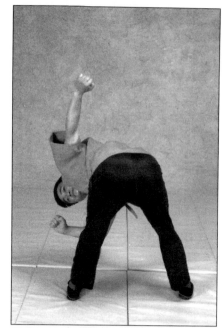

Figure 2-53

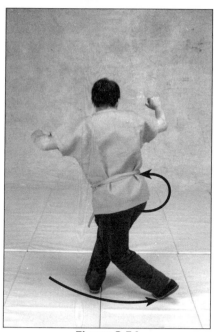

Figure 2-54

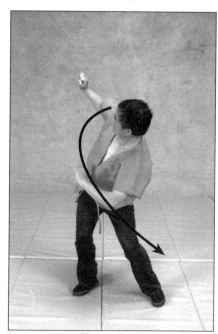

Figure 2-55

3. Fast Entering 快入

Training Method:

This Entering technique is almost exactly the same as the previous techniques **Front Cross Step Entering** and **Back Cross Step Entering** except that from the starting position, you don't step in front or step around behind. Instead you will jump and turn 180 degrees to the left and land with your back facing your opponent

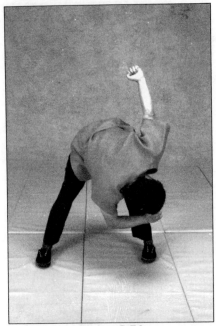

Figure 2-56

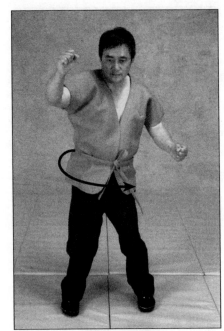

Figure 2-57

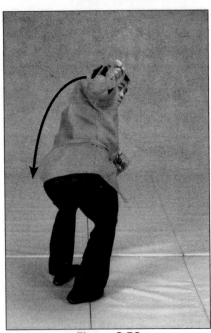

Figure 2-58

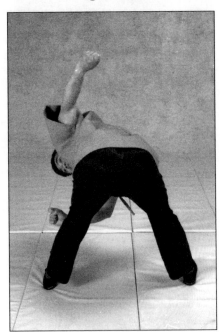

Figure 2-59

in a ready-to-throw posture. After landing, your right hip should thrust against your opponent's lower abdomen. The rest of movements are executed in the same way (Figures 2-57 to 2-59). Train both sides as many times as you like.

4. Carry Entering 攜入

Training Method:

In this technique, you can apply the footwork used in **Front Cross**

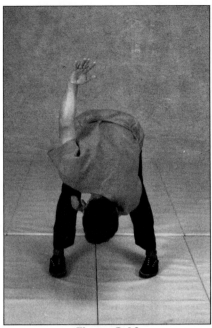

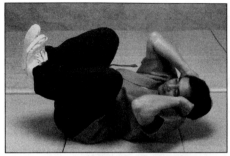

Figure 2-60   Figure 2-61

Step Entering, **Back Cross Step Entering** and **Fast Entering**. The only difference in this technique is that you bend straight forward instead of bending left or right (Figure 2-60).

2-5. Falling 跌法

Training in San Shou Kuai Jiao involves a lot of throwing or being thrown by a partner. In some circumstances, you may need to fall to the ground purposely to execute certain throwing techniques. Therefore, one of the very first skills you need to learn is how to fall. It is of utmost importance that you know how to fall correctly and safely. Being able to fall correctly in any position will help you to prevent injuries. It is also an effective way to train bodily awareness, coordination, and quickness. Another benefit of having good falling skills is that once you have learned and mastered the skill of falling, you will be more relaxed and confident during practice or in a fight.

For all falling training a safety mat is recommended.

1. On Ground Body Position 滾動倒地法

Training Method:

This is a very typical body position used for self protection when you fall. Before you land on the ground, tuck in your chin, contract your body so that the torso is rounded, bend your arms, and use your hands to cover both sides of your head. Land on your side to protect the spine. At the moment of impact, tense up your body by holding your breath to prevent internal organ injury from the force of the landing (Figure 2-61).

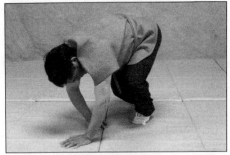

Figure 2-62

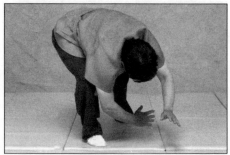

Figure 2-63

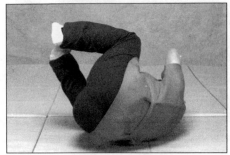

Figure 2-64

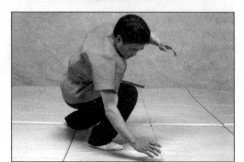

Figure 2-65

2. **Rolling Forward** 搶背

Training Method:

Start with the right foot as the leading foot. Place your right arm at the side of your right foot with fingers pointed inward, and shoulder tucked in. Place your left arm in front of your body, keep your chin tucked in, and the right arm slightly bent with the elbow pointing outwards (Figure 2-62). Roll forward over your right arm, then your shoulder, and then diagonally across the back (Figures 2-63 and 2-64). Repeat the same movement for the left side.

3. **Falling Sideways** 側倒

Training Method:

Start in a squatting position and fall sideways to your right. Before your body makes contact with the ground, keep your right arm bent with fingers pointing inward and use the arm to absorb the shock. Keep your chin tucked in, coil your body, and pull up your knees. Land on your right side (Figures 2-65 and 2-66). Change to the other side and repeat.

4. **Falling Forward** 撐地倒

Training Method:

A). Kneeling Position

Start in a kneeling position with both arms in front of your body

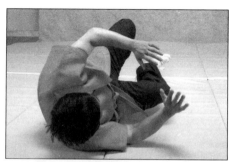

Figure 2-66

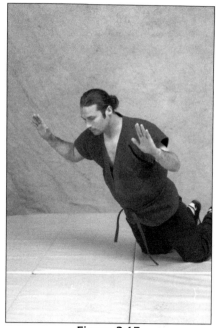

Figure 2-67

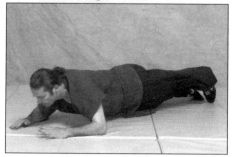

Figure 2-68

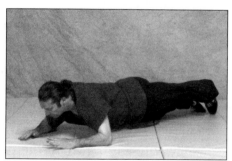

Figure 2-70

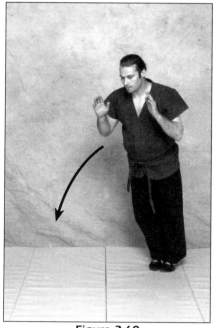

Figure 2-69

and slightly bent (Figure 2-67). Keep your head up and start to fall forward. The palms should make contact first, followed by the forearms to absorb the shock of the fall (Figure 2-68).

B). Standing Position

The degree of difficulty in this position is much greater than the Kneeling Position. You may want to start with the Kneeling Position first, then practice from a Squatting Position and then Standing.

Keep your head up and arms in front of the body. Make contact with the palms and then the forearms (Figures 2-69 and 2-70).

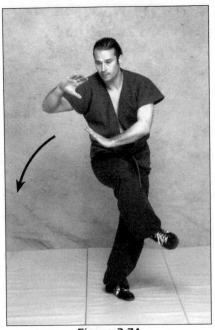

Figure 2-71

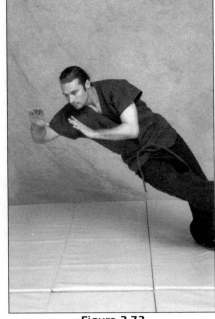

Figure 2-72

5. Coiling Leg and Falling Sideways 屈体盤腿側倒

Training Method:

Coil your right leg upwards, bend your right arm with your palm facing down, bend your left arm in front of the body, and slightly bend your left leg (Figure 2-71).

Fall to the right. The outside of your right leg near the calf should make contact first, then the outside of the thigh. Also use both palms and the inside right forearm to absorb the shock (Figures 2-72 and 2-73).

At the moment of contact, hold your breath and tense up your body. This will help to prevent internal organ damage from the force of the impact.

6. Falling Backward 后倒后背著地

Training Method:

This is a difficult and challenging falling technique. When practicing this falling method, start in a sitting position first, then a squatting position, and finally standing. Also, when practicing from a standing position, you may ask your partner to spot you until you have the confidence to practice on your own. **Be safe**. The falling movement is the same for all positions. We will demonstrate it from a standing position.

Stand up straight with your feet shoulder width apart. Extend both arms to sides as you begin to fall backward (Figure 2-74). As you fall, keep your chin tucked in. Just as the upper part of your

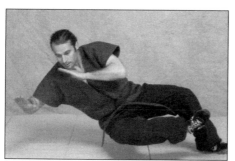

Figure 2-73

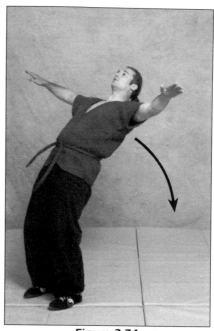

Figure 2-74

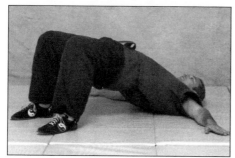

Figure 2-75

back touches the ground, slap the ground with the insides of both arms and thrust your stomach forward (Figure 2-75). Hold your breath and tense your muscles to help prevent injury.

Chapter 3
Basic Training With Equipment

用具基本訓練

3-1. Introduction

Chinese martial arts emphasize basic technique training and body conditioning. It is not hard to understand that body conditioning is necessary for the strength, power and endurance that makes your techniques more powerful. Without basic conditioning, the techniques you learn will not be as effective as they should. There is a saying often heard among Chinese martial artists: "One power suppresses ten techniques" (Yi Li Jiang Shi hui, 一力降十會). It simply means that power can overcome technique. There are different forms of power such as External (Li, physical, muscular) power, Internal (Qi) power, and Mental power. Although there are different forms of power, they are related and it is hard to distinguish between them or separate them one from another.

When applying the throwing techniques of San Shou Kuai Jiao, the power of your hands and arms is very important. Your hands must be able to grab tightly, and your arms should have enough strength and resistance for blocking. When holding or carrying an opponent on your back you need to have power and strength in your waist and legs. The waist and legs need to be strong and flexible in order to make your body movements smooth and swift. When your hands, arms, waist and legs have strength and power, then techniques will become much more effective, and mentally, your confidence will be higher. As a result, you can maximize your fighting ability.

In this chapter, we will introduce some of the traditional equipment training methods to help you to develop the skills and power necessary for San Shou Kuai Jiao techniques. These methods are simple, refined, and very effective for improving the endurance and power of the whole

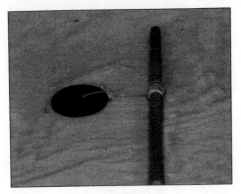

Figure 3-1

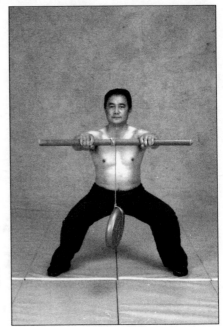

Figure 3-2

body. These training methods, which have been passed down from generation to generation, are necessary if you want to become proficient in San Shou Kuai Jiao. It is impossible to list all the training methods developed for San Shou Kuai Jiao, but the techniques in this chapter will provide you with a strong and well-rounded foundation. If you are interested in other traditional training methods, please refer to the forthcoming traditional Chinese Shuai Jiao book from YMAA Publication Center.

3-2. Body Conditioning With Equipment

1. Windlass 雙手卷棒
To increase the strength and power of the wrists and forearms.

Equipment:
A five to ten pound weight suspended by a cord from the center of a short wooden bar (Figure 3-1).

Training Method:
Squat down in Horse Stance or stand with both feet shoulder width apart. With both hands, hold the bar straight out at shoulder height. Wind the cord onto the bar until the weight reaches the bar. Then unwind the cord to lower the weight. Repeat the exercise and gradually increase the number of repetitions and the amount of weight (Figures 3-2 and 3-3).

2. Single Hand Windlass 單手卷棒
To increase the strength and power of the wrists and forearms. Also increases the grabbing strength of the hands.

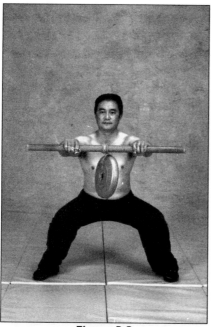

Figure 3-3

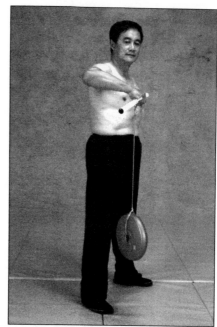

Figure 3-4

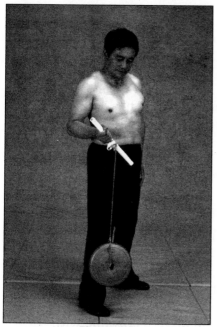

Figure 3-5

Equipment:

A two to six pound weight suspended by a cord from the center of a short wooden bar.

Training Method:

Stand up with both feet shoulder width apart. With one hand grab an end of the bar (Figure 3-4), and turn your wrist so that the other end of the bar will turn counterclockwise in a circular motion (Figure 3-5). Every time you turn the bar downward, it will scoop up the cord and lift the weight (Figure 3-6). Wind the cord onto the bar until the weight is all the way up (Figure 3-7). You must turn your wrist quickly so the cord does not unwind. Repeat the same exercise with the other hand, and gradually increase the number of repetitions and the amount of weight.

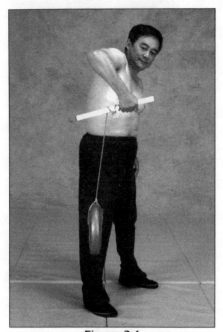

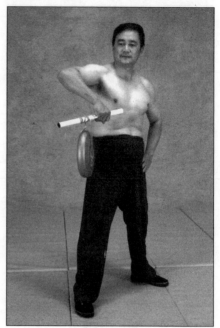

Figure 3-6   Figure 3-7

3. Tossing the Sand Bag 扔沙袋

To increase your squeezing, grabbing, and pulling power. Also to increase body movement coordination.

Equipment:

Use fine canvas to make a bag about 16x16 inches. Fill the bag about one third of the way with sand. Gradually add more sand as your strength increases.

Training Method:

A. SOLO PRACTICE

Tossing Left and Right:

Stand with both feet shoulder width apart and knees slightly bent. With your left hand grab the sand bag at its center (Figure 3-8) and throw it up above your head to your right (Figure 3-9). Then grab the center of the bag with your right hand while it is still in the air. Then throw it up to your left (Figure 3-10). Repeat as many times as you want. When you are comfortable with the exercise, you can add footwork like **Front Cross Step** and **Back Cross Step** while you throw and grab the bag. **Make sure to grab the bag's center.**

Tossing Around the Back:

Stand up with both feet shoulder width apart and your knees slightly bent. With your right hand grab the bag and toss it behind your back and over your head so it will be in front of you to your left. Grab the bag in the air with your left

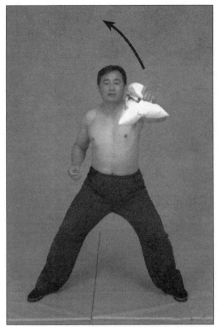

Figure 3-8

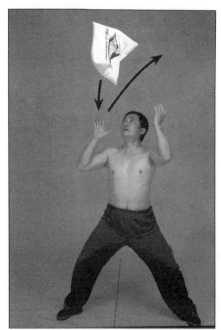

Figure 3-9

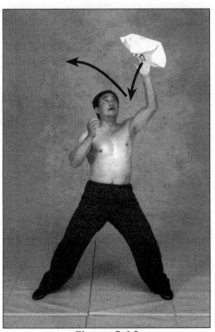

Figure 3-10

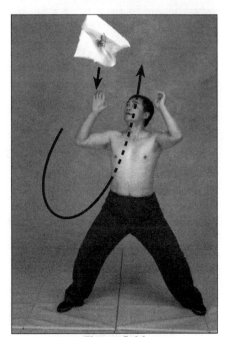

Figure 3-11

hand and toss it to the right over your head so it will be in front of you to your right. Grab the bag with the right hand and repeat the exercise (Figures 3-11 and 3-12). When you are comfortable with this exercise, you can add footwork while you toss and grab the bag.

Tossing Between the Legs:
Stand in Horse Stance. Grab the bag with your right hand

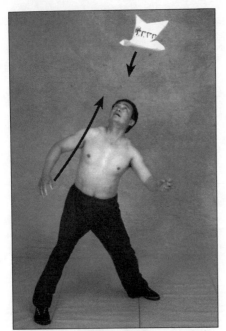

Figure 3-12

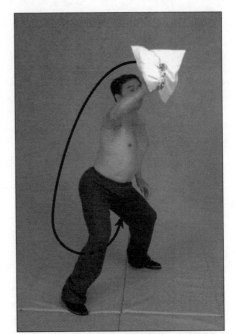

Figure 3-13

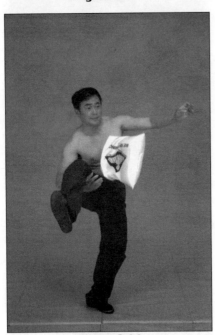

Figure 3-14

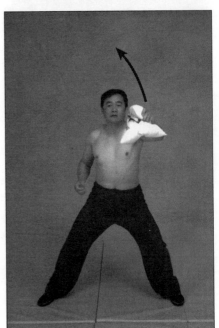

Figure 3-15

and toss it up between both legs from outside of your right leg (Figures 3-13 and 3-14). Grab the bag in the air with the left hand (Figure 3-15) and then toss it up between both legs from the outside of the left leg. Grab the bag with the right hand and repeat the exercise.

B. TWO PERSON EXERCISE:

Two persons face each other. Your partner tosses the bag and you catch it with your right hand. Then toss it up above your

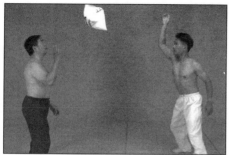

Figure 3-16

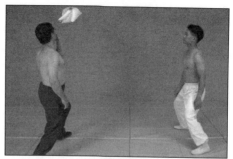

Figure 3-17

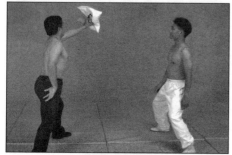

Figure 3-18

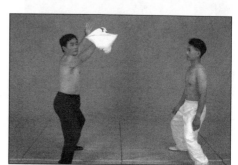

Figure 3-19

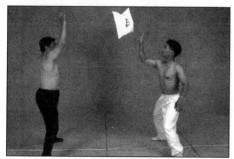

Figure 3-20

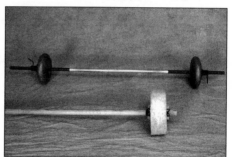

Figure 3-21

head to your left (Figures 3-16 and 3-17). Grab the bag at its center with your left hand while it is still in the air (Figure 3-18). Toss the bag back to your right hand and throw it back to your partner (Figures 3-19 and 3-20). Adjust your distance accordingly. You can throw directly to each other, from behind your back to each other, or between the legs to each other. Be creative and have fun with this exercise.

4. Weight Training 舉重

To increase the strength of the limbs and improve waist power and other powers such as lifting and thrusting through. Also develops body coordination and endurance.

Equipment:

Traditionally, the weight was a stone between 20 and 100 pounds. Modern weight lifting equipment is acceptable (Figure 3-21).

49

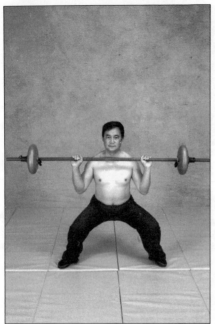

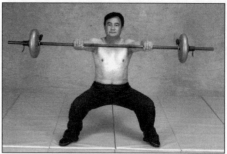

Figure 3-23

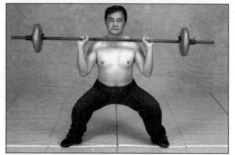

Figure 3-24

Figure 3-22

Training Methods:

A. BOTH HANDS PUSH FORWARD:

Stand in Horse Stance, lift the weight up and push it out in front of your chest at shoulder height (Figures 3-22 and 3-23). Then pull the weight in and repeat as many times as you want (Figure 3-24).

B. WHEELING THE WEIGHT:

Left Side:

Stand up with both feet shoulder width apart and bend slightly at the knees. Hold the weight in front of you with your right palm turned outward and left palm turned inward (Figure 3-25). Back view (Figure 3-26).

Step with your left foot behind and across your right foot (Figure 3-27) and swing the weight upward in a circular motion. Lead with the left hand and pivot 180 degrees, holding the weight above your head (Figure 3-28).

Continuing from Figure 3-28 above, step with your left foot behind and across the right foot and swing the weight downward in a circular motion as you pivot from your waist 180 degrees and back to the original form (Figures 3-29, 3-30, and 3-31). Repeat the exercise and gradually increase the weight and number of repetitions. Be sure that the dumbbells are securely fastened to the bar, and do not swing wildly.

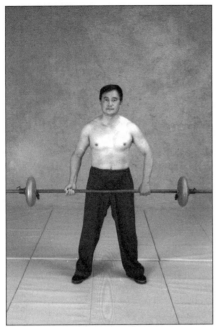

Figure 3-25

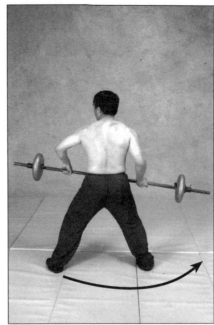

Figure 3-26

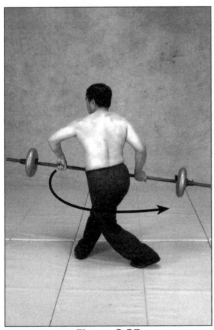

Figure 3-27

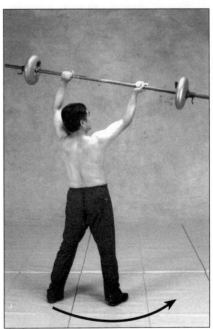

Figure 3-28

Right Side:
Repeat the same exercises in the opposite direction.

5. Pulling Elastic Rope 扯橡皮筋

Pulling elastic rope is another basic of Chinese Wrestling train-ing. It is convenient because you can bring the rope with you to practice where and when you want. This training will help to increase the strength and mobility of the whole body. Elastic

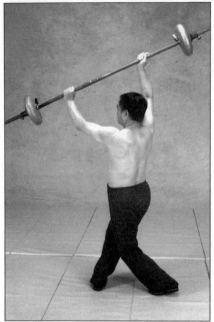

Figure 3-29

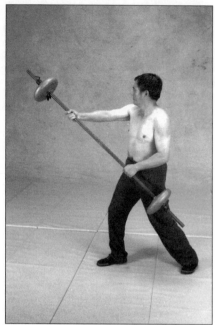

Figure 3-30

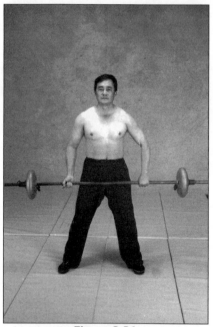

Figure 3-31

rope pulling is often practiced in combination with basic wrestling moves to improve the accuracy and fluency of the techniques.

Equipment:

Traditionally, the equipment consists of pulleys with weights tied at one end of the rope. The weight should vary according to your ability. Elastic rope can also now be used. Tie the rope so that it has one long section joined by two shorter sections. The long section should be two or three times longer. The two shorter sections are for both hands to pull. When practicing, tie the longer end of the rope to a pole or tree. Make sure the rope is secure before using it (Figure 3-32).

Training Method:

A. PULLING SIDEWAYS:

Stand with both feet shoulder width apart. Grab both short ends of the rope in your left hand and stand sideways with your right

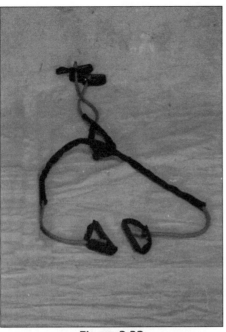

Figure 3-32

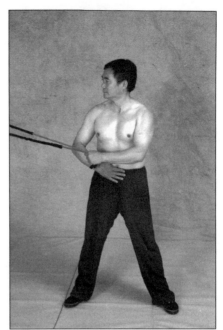

Figure 3-33

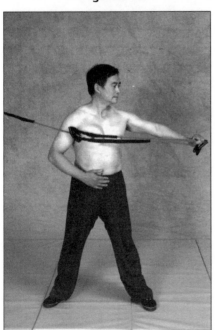

Figure 3-34

shoulder facing the pole (Figure 3-33). Pull the rope in front of you and past your body to your left. Follow the pulling hand with your eyes. Repeat the exercise and gradually increase the number of repetitions. (Figure 3-34).

Change sides and repeat with the right hand.

B. PULLING DOWNWARD SIDEWAYS:

Grab the short ends of the rope with both hands and face the pole with right leg forward (Figure 3-35). Step the right foot across the left foot while pulling the rope down to the left with both hands. Repeat the exercise and gradually increase the number of repetitions. (Figure 3-36).

Change sides and repeat.

C. PULL AND THRUST FORWARD:

Stand with both feet shoulder width apart, grab both ends of the rope with the right hand and face the pole sideways (Figure 3-37).

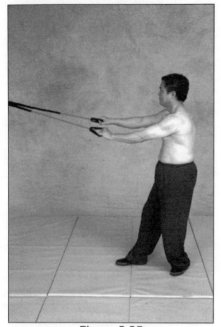

Figure 3-35

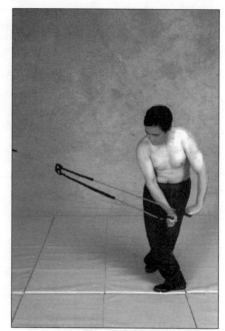

Figure 3-36

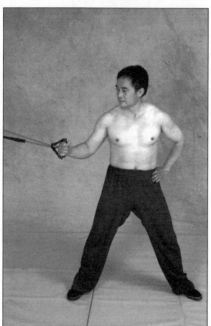

Figure 3-37

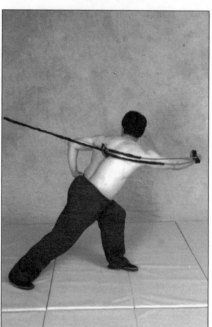

Figure 3-38

Pull the rope to your left in front of you. When it passes your body, twist and push into a Left Bow Stance. The right hand thrusts forward and extends as far as possible while you look back to the left. Repeat the exercise and gradually increase the number of repetitions (Figure 3-38).

Change sides and repeat.

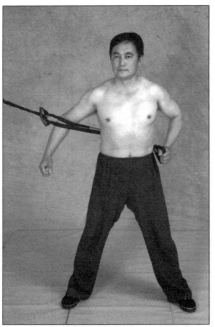

Figure 3-39

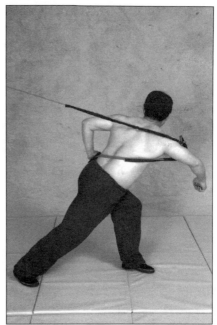

Figure 3-40

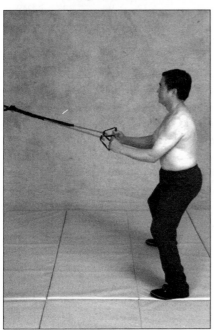

Figure 3-41

D. EXTENDING THE BODY:

Stand with both feet shoulder width apart with the right side of your body facing the pole. Grab both ends of the rope with your left hand and pull it around your back. Hook the rope with your right arm at the inside crook of your elbow (Figure 3-39). Twist your whole body to the left into Left Bow Stance. The right arm pulls forward to the left. Repeat the exercise and gradually increase the number of repetitions (Figure 3-40).

Change sides and repeat.

E. PULLING IN BOTH DIRECTIONS:

Squat down in Horse Stance. Each hand grabs an end of the rope and pulls it in front of you (Figure 3-41). Open the arms out to the sides and then return to the original position (Figures 3-42).

Repeat the exercise and gradually increase the number of repetitions.

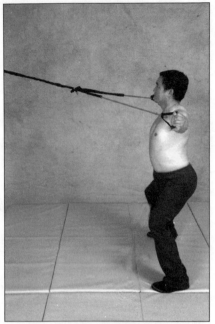

Figure 3-42

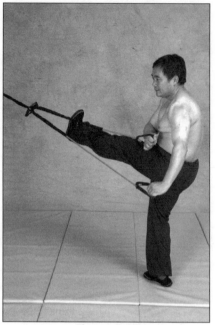

Figure 3-43

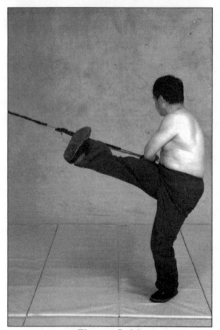

Figure 3-44

F. PULL AND KICK:

Squat down in Horse Stance and grab both ends of the rope, one in each hand. Pull the rope down to your left. Simultaneously kick with the left leg, keeping the toes locked back (Figure 3-43). Change to right side and repeat in the opposite direction (Figure 3-44). While you are kicking, keep the standing leg bent for balance and rooting training.

Repeat the exercise and gradually increase the number of repetitions.

G. LEG HOOKING, BLOCKING TRAINING:

Stand with your right foot forward (Figure 3-45). Grab the ends of the rope with both hands and pull down to your left. Simultaneously, step your left foot behind your right foot (Figure 3-46). Keep pulling the rope and raise both hands in front of your chest (Figure 3-47).

Then twist your body to your left 180 degrees, and kick back and upward in a circular motion with your right leg as high as you can. Keep pulling the rope to your left with your left hand and

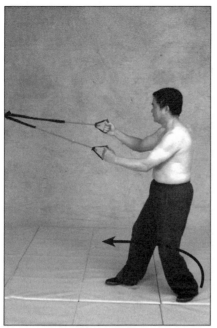

Figure 3-45

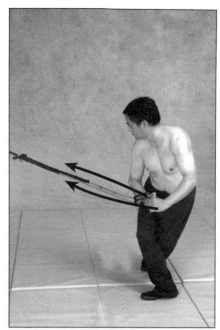

Figure 3-46

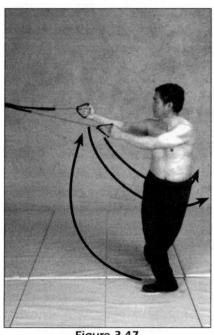

Figure 3-47

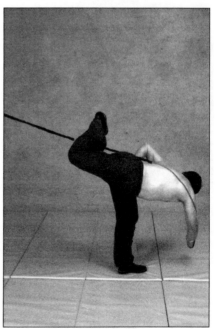

Figure 3-48

with the right hand keep pulling the rope forward then downward in front of you. Your eyes should look back to the left (Figure 3-48). Repeat this exercise as many times as you want.

Change sides and repeat.

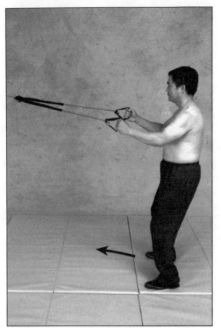

Figure 3-49

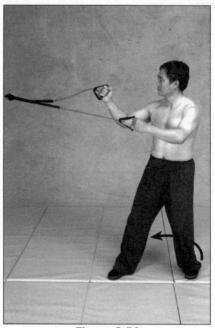

Figure 3-50

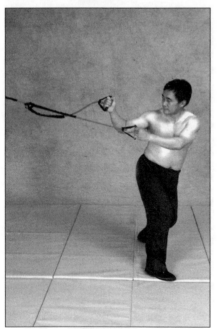

Figure 3-51

H. LOWER LEG BLOCKING, ARMS PULLING AND SHOULDER PRESSING TRAINING:

Face the pole and pull the rope towards you with both hands (Figure 3-49). Step forward with your right foot (Figure 3-50). Step back and around the right foot with your left. Your back should now face the pole (Figure 3-51). Twist and extend your body into a Left Bow Stance and extend your right leg out for a leg block while looking back to your left. Pull the rope upward over your head and then down to your front with your left hand. Simultaneously, pull the rope with your right hand forward to the left (Figure 3-52). Both hands should pull the rope at the same time in a circular motion. Repeat this exercise as many times as you want. Change sides and repeat.

I. FRONT CROSS STEP, CARRYING OVER THE SHOULDER TRAINING:

This is a typical training method for hip throwing techniques. Stand with both legs shoulder width apart and slightly bent. Grab

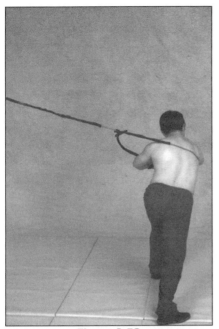

Figure 3-52

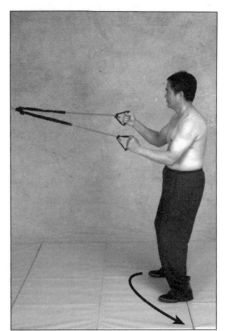

Figure 3-53

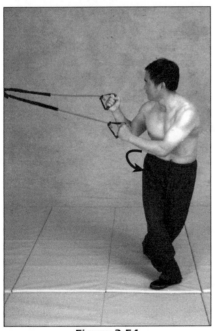

Figure 3-54

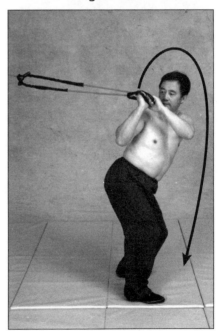

Figure 3-55

the ends of the rope with both hands (Figure 3-53). Step with your right foot across and in front of your left (Figure 3-54). Keeping the legs bent, pivot to the left on the balls of your feet and pull the rope up to your left shoulder (Figure 3-55). Pull the rope down over the shoulder in a circular motion with both hands. Bend at the waist and bow forward deeply. Simultaneously, spring up with both knees. Remember to keep your head tucked in (Figure 3-56).

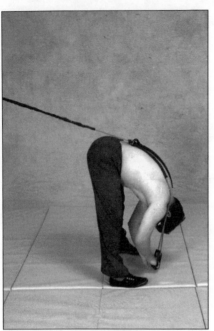

Figure 3-56

Repeat the exercise as many times as you want, and then change sides.

J. BACK CROSS STEP, CARRYING OVER THE SHOULDER TRAINING:

This training is the same as **Front Cross Step, Carrying Over the Shoulder Training** except for the foot work. Instead of stepping in front of the other foot, step across and behind. Feel free to experiment with the foot work when training this exercise.

Chapter 4
Holding Leg(s) Throws

抱腳摔

4-1. Introduction

Holding leg(s) techniques are often used in San Shou Kuai Jiao fighting. They are very effective when defending against an opponent's kicks or for controlling an opponent's leg(s) at close range. These kinds of throws are used when you have the opportunity to hold an opponent's leg(s). Generally, these techniques are used for long range and close range fighting.

In long range fighting these techniques are used when defending against an opponent's kick. Catch or trap the kicking leg and then apply the throw. When applying this type of technique, keep your body as far away from your opponent as possible so that he cannot strike you while you are holding his leg. You need to unbalance your opponent first so that even if he does strike, there will be little power behind it.

For close range fighting, the holding leg(s) techniques require you to get very close to your opponent, and are normally coupled with fakes, attacks, or defenses to disguise your intention. While your opponent is reacting to your first move, you must enter quickly, get hold of his leg(s), unbalance him, then throw him down. Keep in mind that when you are close enough to your opponent to hold his leg(s) you are vulnerable to attack. Therefore, move in and apply the throw as quickly as possible. Avoid struggling with your opponent, and give him no time to react and strike back.

In this chapter, we will introduce San Shou Kuai Jiao techniques for holding an opponent's leg(s) to throw him. Your hold must be tight and strong and the catching, lifting, and pulling movements quick and powerful. The throw itself should also be fast, smooth, and strong. A half-hearted throw is a waste of energy and can put you in a dangerous position.

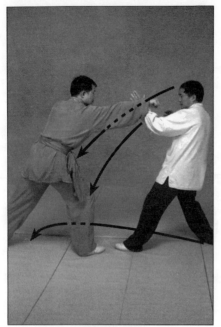

Figure 4-1

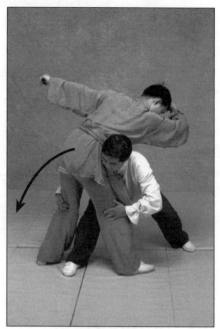

Figure 4-2

4-2. Holding Leg(s) Throwing Techniques

1. Holding Two Legs, Pressing Forward
Throw 抱兩腿前頂摔

a). Gray steps with right foot forward and attacks with a right-handed punch. White blocks outward with his left arm. Then White strikes Gray with both hands to the face or chest (or White will initiate the attack) (Figure 4-1).

b). Gray moves his head to dodge White's attack or raises his arms to block. White moves his hands quickly downward to grab and hold both of Gray's legs. White steps forward with either the right or left foot deep in between Gray's legs (Figure 4-2).

c). White pulls with both hands back and upward with force and drives the body forward, using his shoulder to strike Gray's thigh or abdomen and forcing Gray to fall backward (Figures 4-3 and 4-4).

Key Points

a). Drop low as quickly as possible.

b). Your body weight should be slightly more on the rear leg to create pushing power for the drive. Push forward from the rear leg and lift the hands upward simultaneously.

2. Holding One Leg, Hand Blocking Throw 抱單腿手別

a). Gray's right foot is forward and he attacks with his right hand. White blocks outward with his left arm, then strikes Gray's

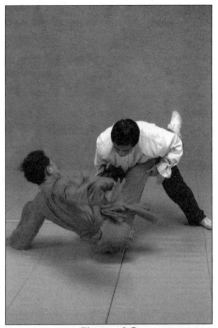

Figure 4-3

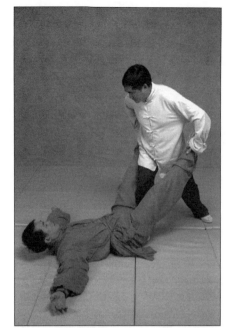

Figure 4-4

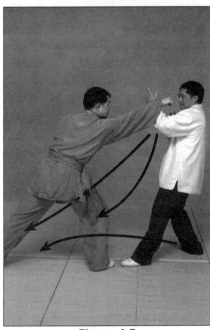

Figure 4-5

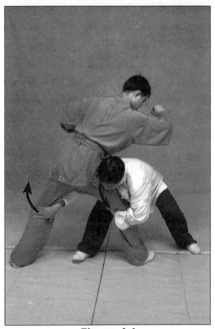

Figure 4-6

face or solar plexus with both hands (or initiates the attack) (Figure 4-5).

b). When Gray moves to dodge the attack or raises his arms to block or swing, White quickly steps his right foot forward deep in between Gray's legs and grabs Gray's right leg. White moves his right hand quickly behind Gray's left leg to block it. White presses firmly on the hollow of Gray's left knee to immobilize him (Figure 4-6).

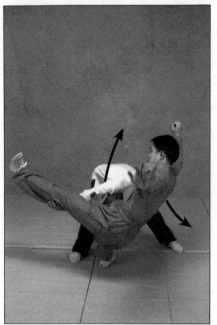

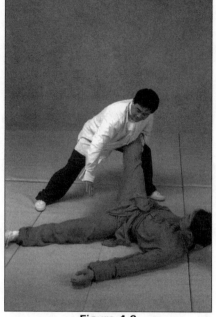

| Figure 4-7 | Figure 4-8 |

c). Then White uses his right shoulder to strike Gray's right thigh and simultaneously turns his body to the left to make Gray fall (Figure 4-7 and 4-8).

Key Points

a). Drop low as quickly as possible. Do not give your opponent time to strike while you are grabbing his legs.

b). Get your front leg as deep as possible in between your opponent's leg.

c). Hold the legs and press firmly with both hands so your opponent can't easily move before the throw is executed.

3. Holding One Leg, Leg Blocking Throw 抱單腿別腿

a). Gray's right foot is forward and he attacks with a right hand strike. White blocks outward with his left arm, then strikes Gray's face or solar plexus with both hands (or initiates an attack) (Figure 4-9).

b). When Gray moves to dodge the attack or raises his arms to block, White takes a half-step forward with his left foot and places it in front of Gray's right foot. White then drops his body and quickly grabs Gray's right leg with his left hand and wraps his right hand around Gray's body. White pivots his left foot outward and extends his right foot in between Gray's legs and behind Gray's left foot (Figure 4-10).

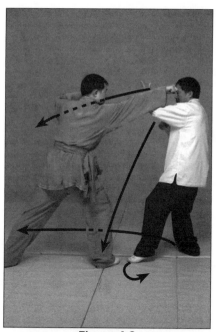
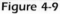

Figure 4-9

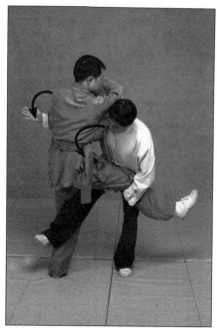

Figure 4-10

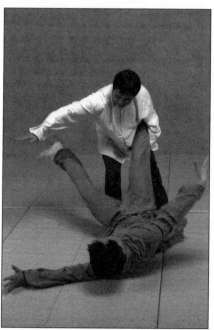

Figure 4-11

c). White twists his body to the left and uses his chest to press Gray's right thigh downward to make Gray fall on his back. Or, White can move forward to make Gray fall backward (Figure 4-11).

Key Points

a). Drop your body and insert your right leg to block your opponent's left foot as quickly as possible.

b). Your left leg should be well bent for good root and balance.

c). When twisting to the left, your right hand and shoulder should also apply force to your opponent's body.

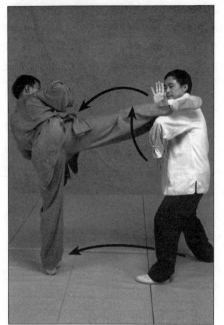

Figure 4-12

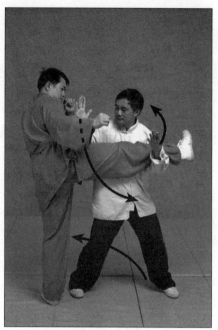

Figure 4-13

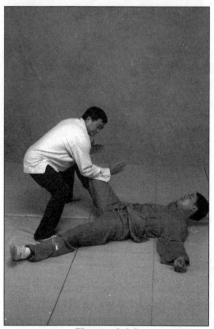

Figure 4-14

4. Holding One Leg, Rotating the Body, Elbow Pressing Throw

摟腿旋身肘壓

a). Gray throws a right round house kick to White's left. White bends his left arm so his elbow points out. White's right arm leans against his upper left arm and the right palm faces outward to block Gray's kick. This is called **Palm and Elbow Crossing Method** (Figure 4-12).

b). White then turns his left hand outward and upward and tightly holds Gray's leg. White steps forward with his right foot and puts it next to Gray's left foot, and uses his right hand to block Gray's right hand (figure 4-13).

c). With his left foot, White steps behind the right leg. White turns quickly to the left and uses his right elbow to press against Gray's thigh to make Gray twist and fall. (Figure 4-14)

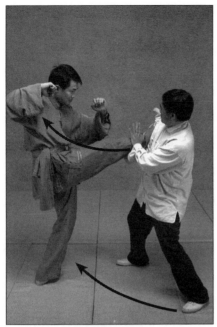

Figure 4-15

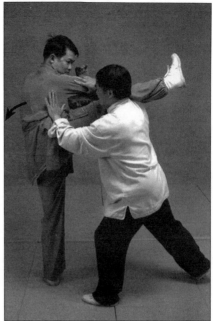

Figure 4-16

Key Points

a). When stepping behind your right foot, keep his right leg tightly locked and pull it towards the rear left corner. Your body weight should be more on the right leg to form a Bow Stance to keep good balance.

b). Your right arm or elbow should press down on your opponent's leg to keep him off balance before the throw.

c). When turning to the left, your body weight should shift from right to left as quickly and smoothly as possible.

5. Holding One Leg, Moving Forward and Pressing Down Throw 摟腿前按摔

a). Gray attacks with a right heel kick or front kick lower than chest height. White is standing with right foot forward. White's right hand moves downward to intercept the kick (Figure 4-15).

b). White steps forward with his left foot while his right hand scoops upward to catch Gray's kicking leg and lock it. White continues to lift with his right arm while his left hand presses on Gray's body to upset Gray's balance (Figure 4-16).

c). White continues to lift and press forward until Gray falls (Figure 4-17).

Key Points

a). Dodge left to evade your opponent's kick before extending your right hand to intercept. This is safer if you miss catching the kicking leg.

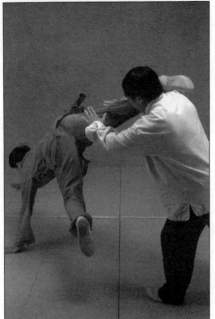

Figure 4-17

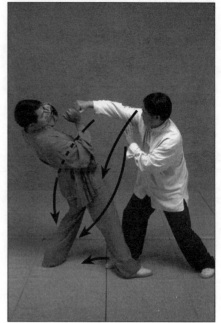

Figure 4-18

6. **Holding Two Legs Sideways Throw** 抱雙腿側摔

a). White initiates the attack with a strike to Gray's head (Figure 4-18).

b). As Gray defends, White drops his body low and steps forward to get closer to Gray. White extends both arms and encircles Gray's legs and holds them tightly against his chest. White then brings his back foot parallel to his front (Figure 4-19).

c). White lifts Gray off the ground and twists to the side to throw Gray down sideways. Alternately, White can first hold Gray's waist, then slide down to grab both legs, lift him up, and throw him sideways (Figure 4-20).

Key points

a). Move quickly to grab and lift your opponent. When squatting down, both knees should be well bent. Snap your knees to lift your opponent.

b). Use your head and shoulder to lean on your opponent's body on the side you want to throw him.

c). The lifting and leaning movements should happen simultaneously.

7. **Holding Two Legs, Backward Throw** 抱雙腿向后摔

a). With his left foot forward Gray attacks with a straight punch to White's head. White ducks to evade the attack (Figure 4-21).

b). White immediately steps forward with his right foot and places

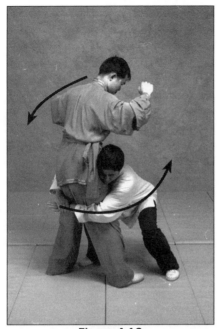

Figure 4-19

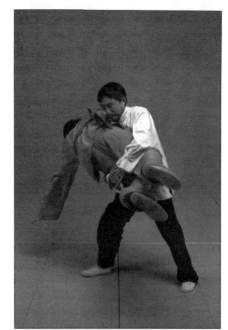

Figure 4-20

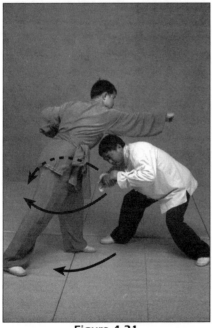

Figure 4-21

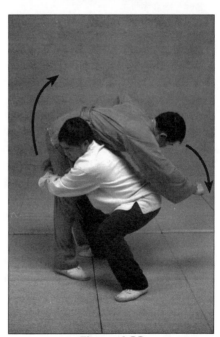

Figure 4-22

it between Gray's legs, then moves his left foot to get closer to Gray. White extends both arms and encircles Gray's legs and holds them tightly against his chest. In the meantime, White puts his right shoulder under Gray's abdomen (Figure 4-22).

c). If Gray leans forward to hold White's back with both of his arms, White immediately holds Gray's legs tightly and straightens up, lifting Gray and throwing him over his shoulder (Figure 4-23).

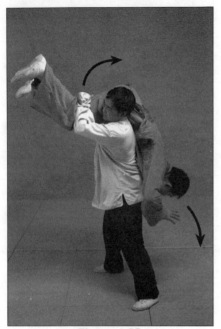

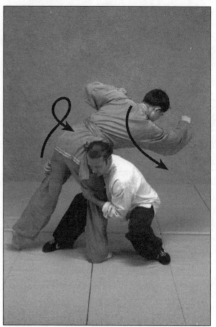

Figure 4-23

Figure 4-24

Key points

a) Before lifting your opponent, both knees should be well bent.

8. Holding Two Legs, Back Falling and Turn Over Throw 抱雙腿后倒翻身摔

a). Gray stands with right foot forward and attacks with a straight punch to the head. White evades the attack and immediately steps forward and places his right foot between Gray's legs. White uses both hands to grab Gray's legs at knee height and puts his right shoulder under Gray's abdomen (Figure 4-24).

b). After grabbing his legs, White continues to straighten up, lifting Gray on his shoulder. White stands and then falls backwards. Once White passes his body's center of gravity, he twists his waist and turns sideways to land on top of Gray (Figure 4-25).

Key points

a). Snap your knees to lift your opponent as high as you can. Hold tightly with both arms when you twist your body sideways.

b). Your opponent should land on his back with you on top. You should twist enough to land chest first instead of back first.

9. Holding and Penetrating Two Legs 抱雙腿黑狗鑽襠

a). Gray holds and presses down on White's shoulders. (Figure 4-26).

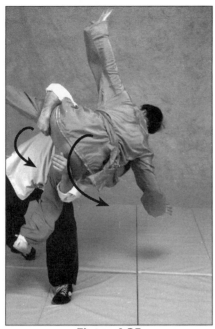

Figure 4-25

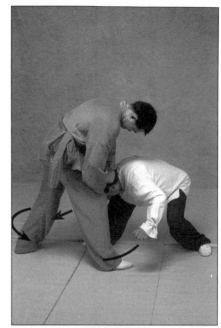

Figure 4-26

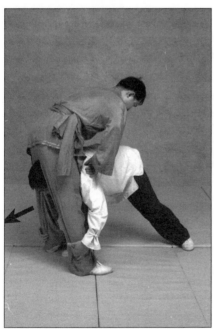

Figure 4-27

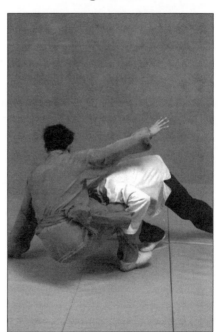

Figure 4-28

b). White takes advantage of being pinned down by diving forward into Gray's legs. White uses both hands to hook and hold both of Gray's ankles from the outside. White then uses his shoulders to press against Gray's lower legs, upsetting his balance (Figure 4-27).

c). White then uses both hands to pull backwards, uprooting Gray and forcing him to fall (Figure 4-28).

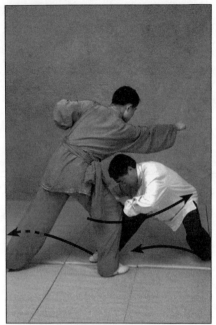

| Figure 4-29 | Figure 4-30 |

Key points

a). Drive your body forward by pushing from your back foot so that your body moves as one unit to maximize the impact on your opponent's legs.

b). Simultaneously press your opponent's legs with your shoulders and pull backwards with your hands.

10. Holding One Leg, Inner Sweeping Throw 抱單腿打腿

a). With his right foot forward Gray attacks with straight punch to the head. White ducks under the punch. White may also initiate the attack and then move in fast while Gray defends (Figure 4-29).

b). White steps forward with his left foot, placing it in front of Gray's right foot. With his left hand White scoops up Gray's right leg and holds it tightly. White extends his right leg between Gray's legs until it reaches the back of Gray's left knee. White presses his right arm against Gray or wraps it around his body. At this point, Gray's weight should be on his left leg (Figure 4-30).

c). Turning to the left, White rolls his right hip forward into Gray's abdomen and swings his right leg backward to strike Gray's supporting leg, throwing Gray to the ground (Figure 4-31).

Key points

a). Your left leg should be well bent and your body should straighten up slightly after your left hand scoops your opponent's right leg.

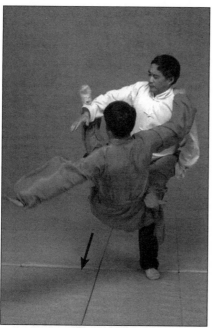

Figure 4-31

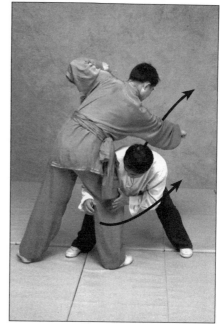

Figure 4-32

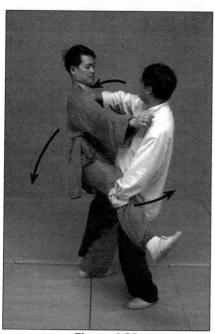

Figure 4-33

b). When sweeping your opponent's leg, your left hand should simultaneously pull to your rear left corner.

11. Holding One Leg, Pushing the Chest Throw

抱單腿推胸摔

a). With his right foot forward Gray attacks with a straight punch to the head. White ducks under the punch. White may also initiate the attack and then move in fast while Gray defends. White lowers his body and grabs Gray's right leg with both hands (Figure 4-32).

b). White steps forward with his left foot and places it in front of Gray's right foot. White lifts Gray's leg with both hands and holds it tightly, then extends his right leg in behind Gray's left foot. White presses with his right hand against Gray's body to upset his balance (Figure 4-33).

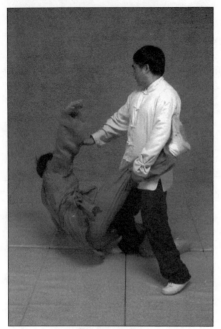

Figure 4-34

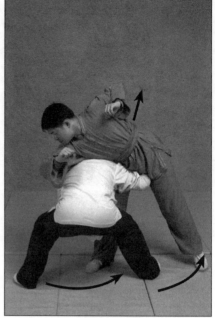

Figure 4-35

c). With his right leg continuing to block Gray's left foot, White pushes forward with his right hand to make Gray fall on his back (Figure 4-34).

Key points

a). Your left leg should be well bent and your body should straighten up slightly after your left hand scoops up your opponent's right leg.

b). Holding One Leg, Pushing the Chest Throw is very similar to #10 except that this technique only uses the right leg to block your opponent's supporting leg and the right hand to push him backward.

12. Holding One Leg, Sideways Throw 抱單腿側拌

a). The holding leg method is same as Figure 4-32 (Figure 4-35).

b). After White grabs Gray's right leg, White makes a half step forward with his left foot to draw near to or parallel with the right foot and uproots Gray. As White lifts his right leg up, White extends his right leg to the outside of Gray's left foot (Figure 4-36).

c). White then sweeps his right foot from right to left. Simultaneously, he uses his head and right shoulder to hit and press sideways to the right to make Gray fall sideways (Figure 4-37).

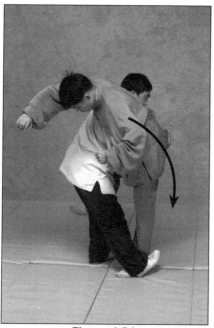

Figure 4-36

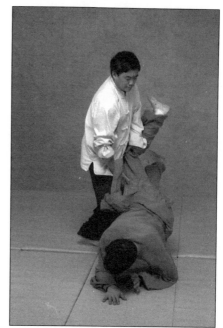

Figure 4-37

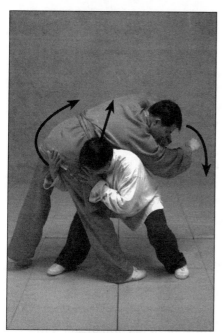

Figure 4-38

Key points

a). Your left leg should be well bent and your body should straighten slightly after lifting your opponent's leg.

b). The foot sweep and the head and shoulder press must be simultaneous.

13. Holding One Leg, Backward Over the Shoulder Throw 抱單腿后摔

a). The holding leg method is the same as figure 4-32, except that after White grabs Gray's right leg, he slips his right hand under Gray's groin area and puts his shoulder under Gray's stomach (Figure 4-38).

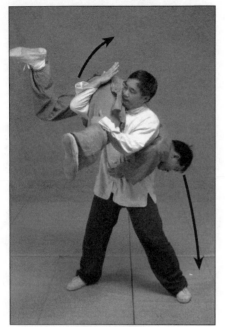

Figure 4-39

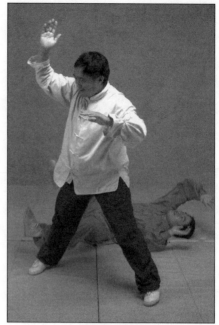

Figure 4-40

b). White straightens up and throws Gray over his shoulder (Figures 4-39 and 4-40).

Key points

a). Both knees should be well bent when you squat down. Snap both legs and straighten your waist when you stand. Your right arm should lift upwards to your back.

14. Holding One Leg, Lifting Up Throw 抱單腿上托

a). Gray attacks with a front kick or heel kick at White's torso. White leans back slightly or steps back to evade the kick. White uses both hands to catch Gray by the ankle (Figure 4-41).

b). White lifts Gray's foot and pushes forward to make him fall (Figure 4-42 and 4-43).

Key points

a). You must lift fast to catch your opponent by surprise. This will give him no time to pull his leg back. Remember to push your opponent's leg forward toward his body while lifting.

15. Holding One Leg, Pulling Throw 抱單腿下拉

a). Gray attacks with a front kick or heel kick to White's torso. White uses both hands to catch Gray's kick at the ankle (Figure 4-44).

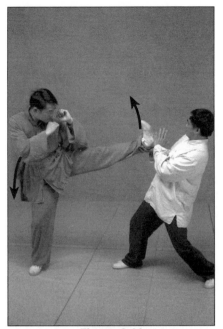

Figure 4-41

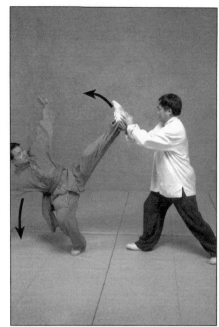

Figure 4-42

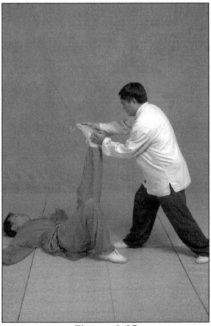

Figure 4-43

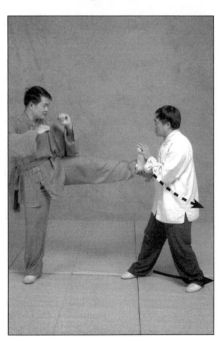

Figure 4-44

b). White, holding the ankle with both hands, steps back with his front foot and jerks Gray's leg forward and downward with strength and speed to make Gray fall (Figure 4-45).

Key points

a). Your back step should be as long as possible. Give your opponent no time to pull back.

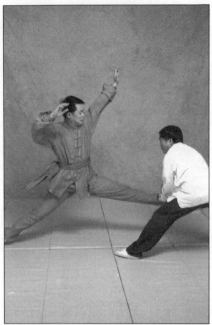

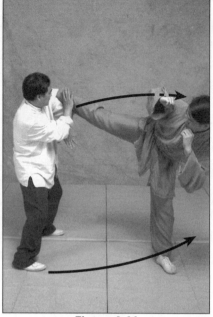

| Figure 4-45 | Figure 4-46 |

16. Holding One Leg, Pressing the Neck Throw

抱單腿壓頸勾腿

a). Gray throws a right roundhouse kick to White's left side. White uses the **Palm and Elbow Crossing Method** to block Gray's kick (Figure 4-46).

b). White holds Gray's right lower leg with his left hand, and extends his right hand to the back of Gray's neck and presses downward. Simultaneously, White extends his right foot to hook and kick Gray's supporting left leg (Figure 4-47).

c). White turns his body to the rear right while his hand keeps pressing downward to destroy Gray's balance. White's right leg continues the hooking motion to make Gray fall (Figure 4-48).

Key points

a). Your left leg should stay slightly bent to maintain good balance throughout the throw.

b). Apply force simultaneously when hooking your opponent's supporting leg and pressing with your hand.

c). Adjust the distance between you and your opponent accordingly so that you can hook his leg.

17. Holding One Leg, Hooking and Pushing

Forward Throw 抱單腿摟踢前推

a). Gray throws a right roundhouse kick to White's left side. White uses the **Palm and Elbow Crossing Method** to catch and hold Gray's left leg with his left arm (Figure 4-49).

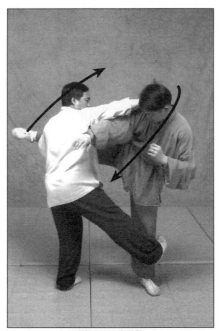

Figure 4-47

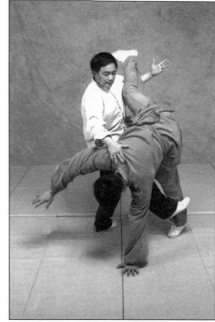

Figure 4-48

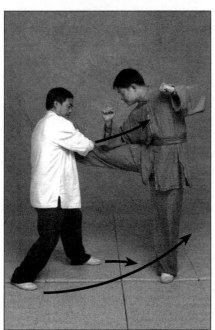

Figure 4-49

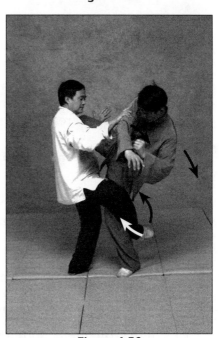

Figure 4-50

b). White steps forward with his left foot, then extends his right leg to the outside of Gray's left leg and hooks behind the knee. With his right hand, White pushes forward and downward on Gray's shoulder to upset his balance (Figure 4-50).

c). White continues to lift with his left arm and apply force with his right hand. White hooks his right leg toward himself to throw Gray down (Figure 4-51).

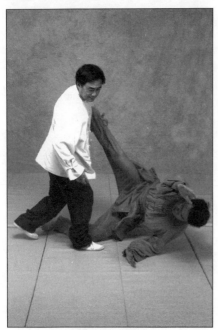

| Figure 4-51 | Figure 4-52 |

Key points

a). Your left leg should be well bent to keep good balance at all times.

b). After hooking your opponent's leg, pull it closer to you to upset his balance. The right leg must coordinate with the right hand to create symmetry power for a strong takedown.

18. Holding One Leg, Carrying Over the Shoulder Throw

抱單腿過背

a) Gray attacks with a right heel kick to White's torso. White, with right foot forward, catches Gray's kicking leg with both hands. (Figure 4-52).

b). White steps sideways with his left leg behind the right, turns his body counterclockwise on the ball of his right foot and squats down with his back facing Gray. At the same time, White pulls Gray's leg onto his right shoulder (Figure 4-53).

c). White straightens both legs slightly and pulls Gray's leg over then inward to his stomach. White keeps his chin tucked in and bends forward to throw Gray over his shoulder (Figure 4-54).

Key points

a). Both knees should be well bent.

b). Pull your opponent's leg forward and into your stomach as quickly and forcefully as possible so he doesn't have time to stabilize himself.

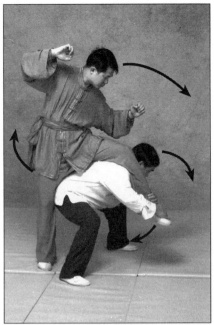

Figure 4-53

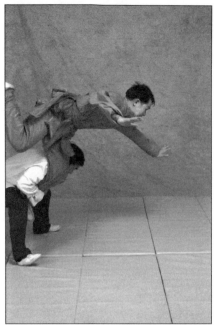

Figure 4-54

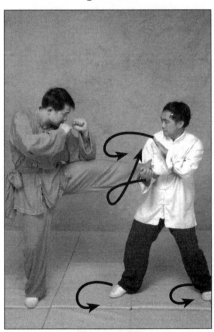

Figure 4-55

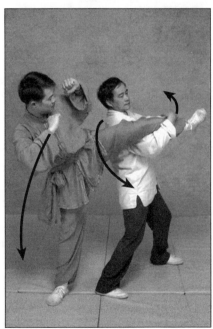

Figure 4-56

19. Scooping the Leg, Shoulder Pressing Throw 抄腿掀靠

a). Gray attacks with a left heel kick to White's midsection. White moves to the right to evade the kick and catches Gray's leg at the same time with a right-handed scoop (Figure 4-55).

b). White continues to raise his right hand while turning to the left. Simultaneously White uses his right shoulder to strike Gray's left thigh. White steps back with his right foot after his

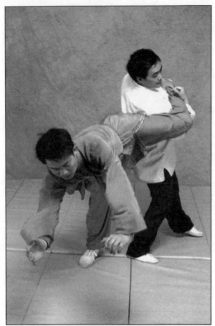

Figure 4-57

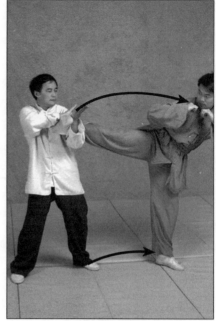

Figure 4-58

body turns to the left. This reinforces the stability for the shoulder strike (Figure 4-56).

c). White uses both hands to hold Gray's left leg and keeps turning left. His right shoulder keeps pressing Gray's left leg to make him fall (Figure 4-57).

Key Points

a). Slide your right foot backwards and twist your body to your left as quickly as possible.

20. Holding the Leg, Pushing the Shoulder Throw

摟腿推胸

a). Gray attacks with a right heel kick or side kick to White's midsection. White moves left and scoops down with his left hand to catch Gray's leg and hold it tightly (Figure 4-58).

b). White steps forward with his left foot and hooks Gray's left ankle while using his right hand to push Gray's shoulder to make Gray fall sideways (Figure 4-59 and 4-60).

Key Points

a). When stepping forward with your left foot, be ready for a possible right-handed strike from your opponent. An option is to seal your opponent's right elbow before coming in.

b). Use your back foot to drive forward to create pushing momentum for more power.

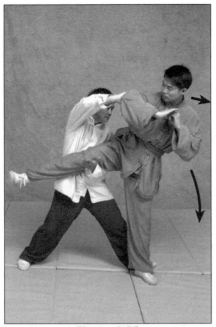

Figure 4-59

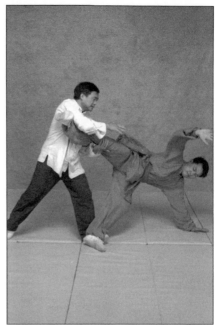

Figure 4-60

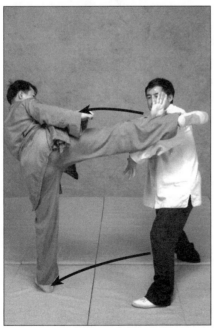

Figure 4-61

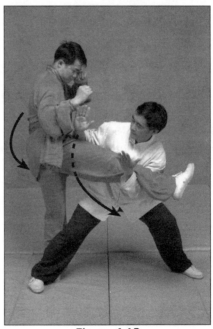

Figure 4-62

21. Holding and Checking Leg Throw 摟腿挫壓

a). Gray throws a right roundhouse kick to White's left side. White intercepts with the **Palm and Elbow Crossing Method** (Figure 4-61).

b). White then turns his left hand outward and then upward to hold Gray's right leg tightly. White extends his right leg to the back of Gray's left ankle to block his foot. White strikes with

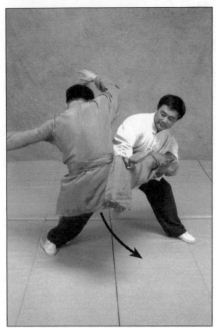

Figure 4-63

his right hand and presses forward or seals Gray's right hand to prevent him from striking (Figure 4-62).

c). White continues to hold Gray's right leg. White uses his right hand to keep pressing forward and down to the left. White twists quickly to the left to throw Gray down (Figure 4-63).

Key Points

a). After catching your opponent's leg, hold it tightly and bring it close to your body so that when you twist to the left, you can also use your body weight to press his leg to make him fall.

b). Twist your body to the left as quickly as possible and sink low to keep good balance.

Chapter 5

Over the Back/Holding the Waist Throwing Methods

過背抱腰摔

5-1. Introduction

The goal of San Shou Kuai Jiao techniques is to disable your enemy's fighting ability as quickly as you can. To achieve this, you need to throw your opponent as hard as possible. However, the opportunity to throw your opponent to the ground does not come often in a fight, because you and your opponent's body positions change constantly. You need to react to the changes and be able to improvise so that you can apply similar types of techniques but use them differently to achieve the takedown. In any case, success depends on the situation and opportunity. There is no best throw. The technique that works for you is the best technique at that time.

In this chapter, we will introduce two different types of throwing techniques. The first type is **Over the Back Throwing Methods**, which have very high combat value and are often used in fighting. In these types of throws, your back is to your opponent and you rely on the coordination of the hips, arms and legs to throw your opponent high over your back or shoulder. These kinds of techniques are extremely useful against an opponent who doesn't know how to fall. If you do not know how to fall, it is natural that you will panic while you are in the air and have no control over your own body. Falling incorrectly can cause devastating injury to the body.

The second type is **Holding the Waist Throwing Methods**. With this type of throw you use your arms to hold an opponent's waist and then lift him up to throw him, or to upset his balance for a takedown. This

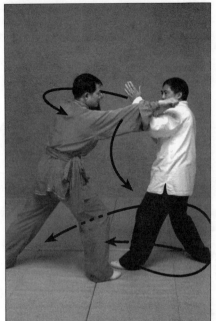

Figure 5-1

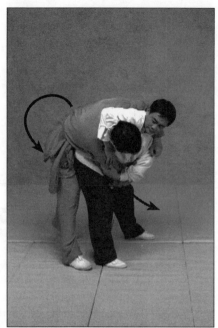

Figure 5-2

kind of throwing technique is best suited for a shorter person with a low center of gravity. Of course, strong arms and legs are also a help.

5-2. Over the Back Throwing Methods 過背摔法

1. Squeezing the Neck, Hip Throw 夾脖揹摔

a). With his right foot forward Gray attacks with his right hand. White blocks the punch with his left forearm, presses downward and tightly grabs Gray's upper arm (Figure 5-1).

b). White then steps forward and, using the ball of the right foot to pivot to the left, steps inside Gray. White's heels are now parallel in front of Gray's feet, with both knees slightly bent in a high Horse Stance. White presses his buttocks tightly against Gray's abdomen. At the same time he uses his right arm to lock Gray's neck (Figure 5-2).

c). White snaps his upper body upward to the left and bends forward with body momentum. Simultaneously, he pulls Gray downward and to the left with the arm and neck lock. By coordinating the waist, buttocks, and the pulling of both arms, White uproots Gray and throws him over his back to the ground (Figures 5-3 and 5-4).

Key Points

a). Both knees should be bent for good root and balance.

b). Your left hand should keep pulling your opponent's right arm throughout the throw.

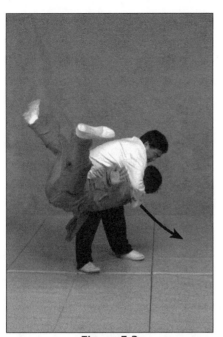

Figure 5-3

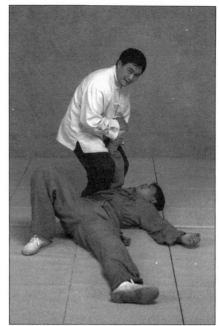

Figure 5-4

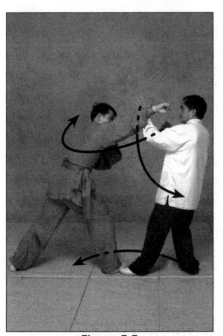

Figure 5-5

2. Lifting the Arm, Holding the Shoulder, Over the Back Throw 插腋抱肩過背摔

a). Gray attacks with a right hook to White's head. White steps forward with his left foot and blocks the punch with his left arm from left to right (Figure 5-5).

b). White steps forward with his right foot and puts it between Gray's feet. At the same time he thrusts his right hand into Gray's right armpit and lifts upward. White uses his left hand to grab Gray's right upper arm or clothing and pull downward into White's chest. At this point Gray should be leaning forward to his right (Figure 5-6).

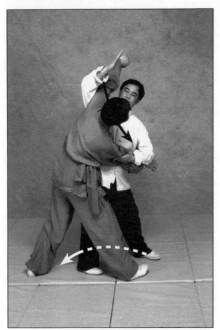

Figure 5-6

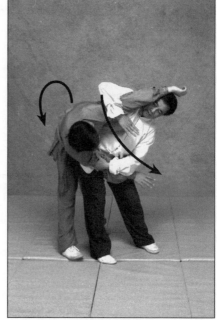

Figure 5-7

c). White steps his left foot behind his right foot and turns to the left into a high Horse Stance. Both feet are parallel and in front of Gray's feet. White's back is now to Gray and his right buttock presses against Gray's abdomen. White twists to the left and makes a circular, downward motion with his right hand to keep Gray's left arm stretched out (Figure 5-7).

d). Simultaneously, White's knees spring up while his left hand keeps pulling Gray's right arm. White moves his body and keeps lifting with his right arm and hip so that Gray is pulled over his back (Figure 5-8).

Key Points

a). Always keep your opponent's body close against your right hip.

b). Both arms should make circular motions when pulling your opponent down.

3. Holding the Waist, Over the Back Throw 抱腰過背摔

a). Gray attacks with right punch to the head. White dodges right, steps forward with his left foot, and blocks the punch with his left arm (Figure 5-9).

b). White steps forward with his right foot and puts it in between Gray's feet. Simultaneously, White moves his right hand under Gray's right arm to hold Gray's waist. With his left hand White then grabs Gray's right hand and pulls it downward close to his body (Figure 5-10).

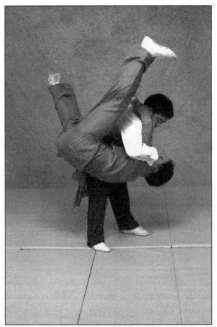

Figure 5-8

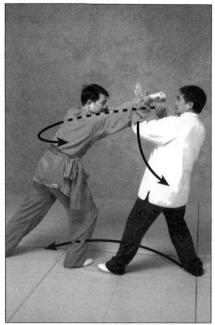

Figure 5-9

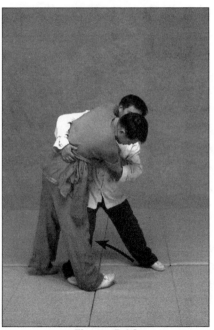

Figure 5-10

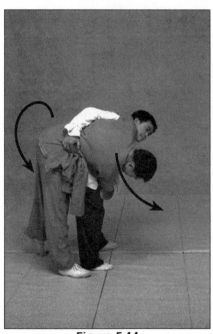

Figure 5-11

c). White steps his left foot behind his right foot and turns to the left into a high Horse Stance, knees bent. Both feet are parallel, and White's back faces Gray while his buttocks press against Gray's abdomen (Figure 5-11).

d). Keeping his head tucked in, White springs up with the knees, lifting Gray with his hip and pulling Gray with his left hand.

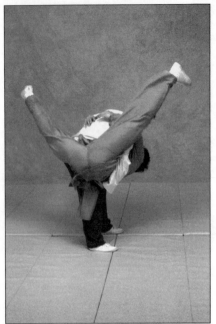

Figure 5-12

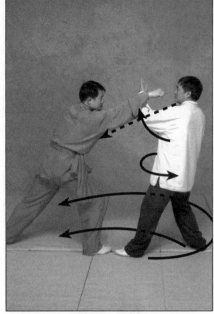

Figure 5-13

Still holding Gray's waist White twists his body to throw Gray over his back (Figure 5-12).

Key Points

a). This technique is very similar to technique #2 except that your right arm holds your opponent's waist instead of lifting his right arm upward.

4. **Penetrating and Holding the Arm, Over the Back Throw** 穿臂抱臂過背摔

a). Gray attacks with a right punch to the head. White dodges right and blocks and grabs the punch with his left arm (Figure 5-13).

b). White then reaches with his right hand to grab and hold Gray's right arm while pulling with the left. Simultaneously, White steps his right foot forward and his left foot behind and around the right foot into Horse Stance, knees deeply bent. Both feet are parallel, and White's buttocks press against Gray's abdomen (Figure 5-14).

c). Keeping his head tucked in and springing up with straight knees, White lifts and throws Gray over his back (Figure 5-15).

Key Points

a). After entering the throwing position, both hands should pull continuously on your opponent's right arm to upset his balance.

b). Keep both knees deeply bent and keep your body close to your opponent's.

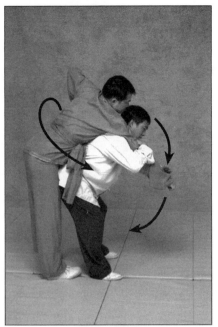

Figure 5-14

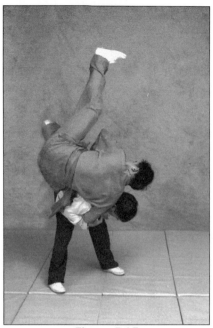

Figure 5-15

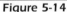

5. Squeezing the Neck, Sweeping the Leg, Over the Back
Throw 夾頸向后打腿過背摔

a). Gray's stance is right foot forward and he attacks with a right punch to the head. White blocks the punch and grabs it with his left hand (Figure 5-16).

b). White wraps up Gray's neck with his right arm while his left hand pulls Gray's arm to the left. At the same time White steps his left foot forward and places it in front of Gray's right foot. White then pivots on his left foot to his left and slides his right leg outside Gray's right leg, while pulling Gray close against his body. Now Gray's weight is on his right leg and slightly forward, upsetting his balance (Figure 5-17).

c). White twists to the left and simultaneously sweeps upward with his right leg. White's left hand pulls Gray's right arm downward and to the left to throw him down (Figure 5-18).

Key Points

a). Keep your left leg bent and your upper body turned slightly to the right to set up for the throw.

b). As you twist to your left, kick back as high as possible with the right leg. This will sweep your opponent's legs high off the ground and make him fall on his back.

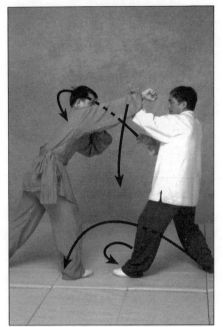

Figure 5-16

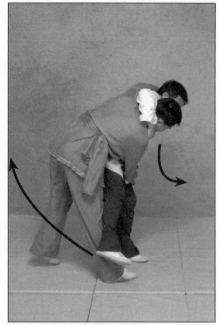

Figure 5-17

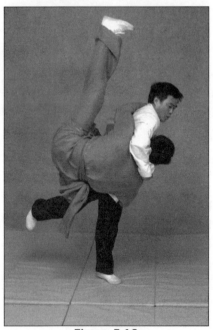

Figure 5-18

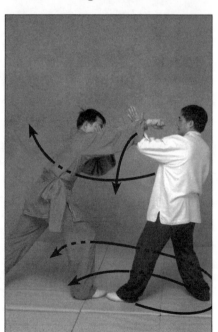

Figure 5-19

6. **Lifting the Arm, Holding the Shoulder, Sweeping the Leg, Over the Back Throw** 插腋抱肩向后打腿過背摔

   a). With his right foot forward, Gray attacks with a right punch to the head. White blocks the punch and grabs it with his left hand (Figure 5-19).

   b). White thrusts his right arm under Gray's left armpit to lock his shoulder and scoop it up. With his left hand White grabs

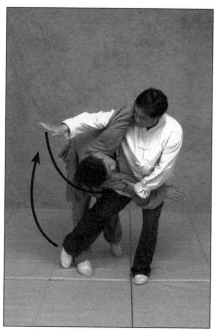

Figure 5-20

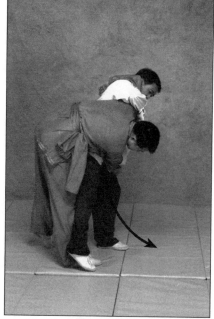

Figure 5-21

Gray's right arm and pulls it to the left. At the same time, White pivots to the left on his left foot and slips his right leg outside Gray's right leg, and pulls Gray close against his body. Now Gray is leaning forward slightly and losing his balance (Figure 5-20).

c). White twists to the left and simultaneously sweeps upward with his right leg. White continues to pull Gray's right arm downward and to the left and uses his right hand to keep pressing downward to the left to throw Gray (Figure 5-21).

Key Points

a). Similar to Technique #5 except that your right hand goes under your opponent's right shoulder instead of locking your opponent's head.

5-3. Holding the Waist Throwing Methods 抱腰摔法

1. Holding the Waist, Falling Back and Turning Over Throw
抱腰后倒翻身摔

a). Gray attacks with a right punch to the head. White protects his head with both hands and dodges to the right. White quickly steps forward to hold Gray's waist with both arms and puts his right shoulder under Gray's abdomen (Figures 5-22 and 5-23).

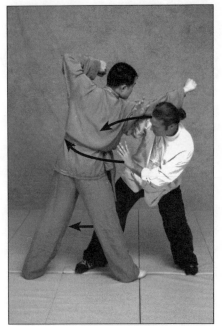

Figure 5-22

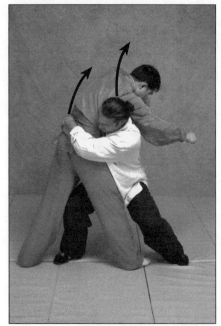

Figure 5-23

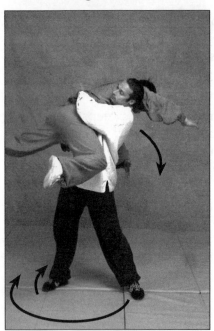

Figure 5-24

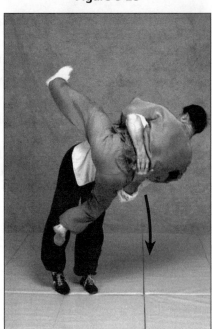

Figure 5-25

b). White straightens his knees to lift Gray, bends backward, keeps his head face up and begins to fall backward. While still falling, he turns over just before his head touches the ground to land on top of Gray (Figures 5-24 and 5-25).

Key Points

a). If you are carrying your opponent on your right shoulder, fall backward and turn your body to your right. Turn to the left if you are carrying him on your left shoulder.

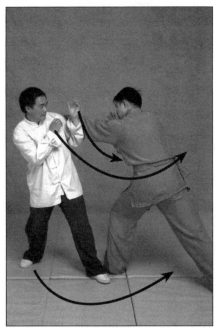

Figure 5-26

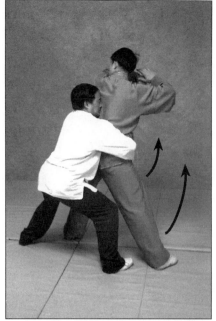

Figure 5-27

b). When falling, your opponent's head and shoulder should hit the ground first. Follow up by landing on top of him with your body.

2. Holding the Waist From Behind Throw 后抱腰摔

a). Gray attacks with a left punch to the head. White blocks with his left arm and steps his left foot forward, placing it outside of Gray's left foot (Figure 5-26).

b). White then steps forward and around with his right foot and places it behind Gray's right. He then reaches with his right hand behind Gray's back and grabs Gray's waist with both arms (Figure 5-27).

c). White holds tightly and lifts. With Gray off the ground, White leans to his right and turns both arms like a steering wheel to throw Gray down (Figures 5-28 and 5-29).

Key Points

a). Bend both knees and hold your opponent tight and close.

b). Spring up with the knees to lift your opponent as high as possible off the ground.

c). Turn both arms clockwise or counterclockwise to throw your opponent sideways.

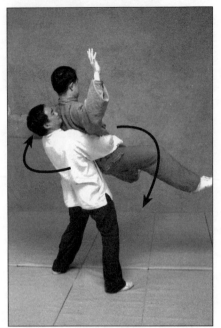

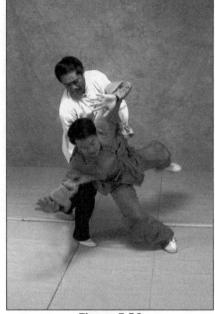

Figure 5-28   Figure 5-29

3. Holding the Waist From Behind, Falling Backward Throw 后抱腰后倒翻身摔

a). Gray attacks with a left punch to the head. White blocks with his left arm, steps his left foot forward and places it outside of Gray's left foot (Figure 5-30).

b). White steps his right foot forward and around and places it behind Gray's right foot. He then reaches his right hand behind Gray's back and holds his waist with both arms (Figure 5-31).

c). White holds tightly and lifts Gray. He leans backward slightly with his head facing up and falls backwards. At this point, Gray should lose all his balance and control (Figure 5-32).

d). Just as White's head is about to hit the ground he twists his body to the left . Gray hits the ground chest first and White lands on top (Figure 5-33).

Key Points

a). Bend both knees deeply and hold your opponent's body tight and close to you.

b). Spring up from both knees to lift your opponent as high as possible.

c). The timing of the fall and the body twist are important for a successful throw.

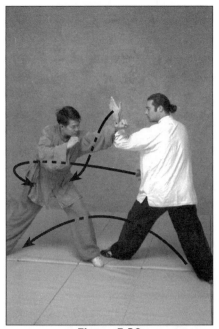

Figure 5-30

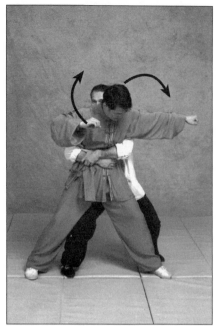

Figure 5-31

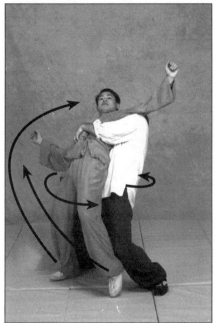

Figure 5-32

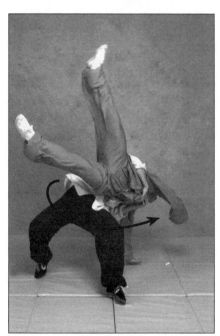

Figure 5-33

4. Holding the Waist, Winding the Leg, Pressing Forward Throw 抱腰盤腿前壓

a). With his right foot forward, Gray attacks with a left punch to the head. White blocks it with his left hand (Figure 5-34).

b). White steps forward and puts his right foot between Gray's feet, dodges downward and reaches with both hands behind Gray's back to hold his waist (Figure 5-35).

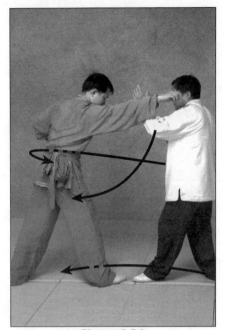

Figure 5-34

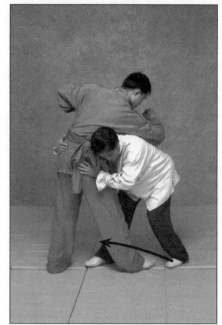

Figure 5-35

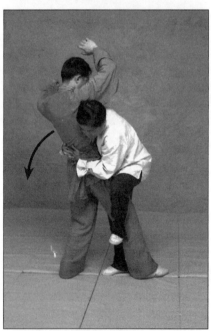

Figure 5-36

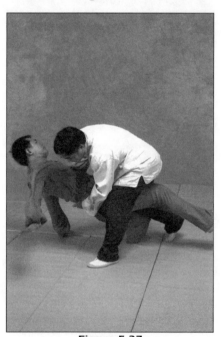

Figure 5-37

c). White then places his left foot outside Gray's right leg. He uses his left leg to wrap Gray's right leg, hook it up and pull it backward. White then stands up slightly so that his right shoulder is under Gray's armpit to prevent Gray from elbowing him. White pulls Gray toward him and holds tightly (Figure 5-36).

d). Simultaneously, White uses his upper body to press forward against Gray's chest, making him fall on his back (Figure 5-37).

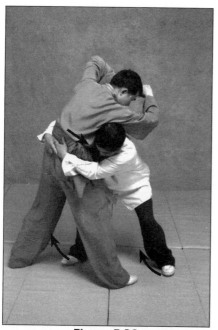

Figure 5-38

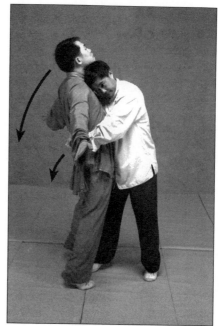

Figure 5-39

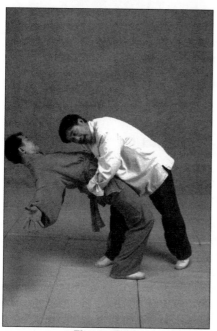

Figure 5-40

Key Points

a). Bend your right knee deeply to keep good root and balance.

b). When landing, you can use your shoulder to strike your opponent, or put a knee in his groin.

5. Strangle the Waist, Leap Up, and Strike with Head Throw 砸腰跳起頭撞摔

a). White gets inside Gray's guard to hold Gray's waist with both arms (Figure 5-38).

b). White squeezes tightly and pulls Gray's waist close to his body while leaning forward. This upsets Gray's balance. White brings his rear foot closer to the front foot and springs up on both legs to smash Gray's face or lower cheekbone with his head. Then White pushes forward to make Gray fall backward to the ground (Figures 5-39 and 5-40).

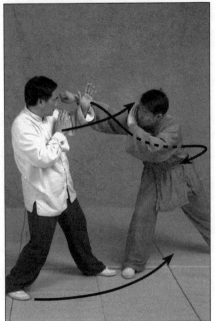

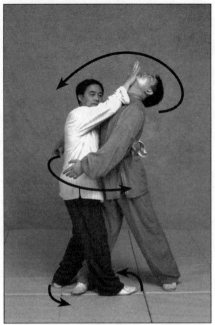

Figure 5-41  **Figure 5-42**

Key Points

a). Hold your opponent's waist or back tightly and close to your body throughout the execution of the technique.

b). After the head strike, use your head and chest to push forward.

6. Holding the Waist, Pushing the Chin and Rotating the Body Throw 抱腰推頤旋身摔

a). With his right foot forward Gray attacks with a right punch to the head. White blocks it with his left arm (Figure 5-41).

b). White steps his right foot forward and puts it in between Gray's feet and quickly gets his left hand behind Gray's back. White shoots his right hand forward to push Gray's chin upward and back (Figure 5-42).

c). White then pivots his right foot to the left while his left foot makes a small step to the right. This puts him in better position to upset Gray's balance. White holds Gray's waist tightly and draws it close to his body while pushing Gray's chin upwards. At this point, Gray should be leaning back with his weight on his right leg (Figure 5-43).

d). White pushes Gray's chin forward and then downward to the left to make Gray fall on his back (Figure 5-44).

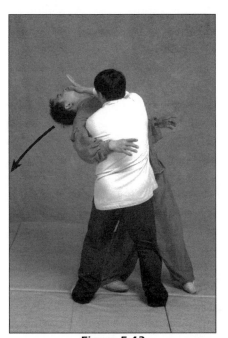

Figure 5-43

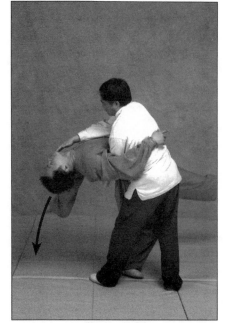

Figure 5-44

Key Points

a). The rotation of your body must coordinate with your left hand, which is drawing your opponent's waist close to you. Apply pressure with your right hand and extend forward and then downward to make the throw successful.

Chapter 6
Leg Hooking Throws

勾腳摔

6-1. Introduction

Leg hooking is a major technique used in San Shou Kuai Jiao. It is very effective and minimizes the use of energy to take down an opponent. Also, leg hooks are hard to detect in close range situations because fighters tend to pay more attention to an opponent's hands. If you can distract your opponent with your hands, or if you have the opportunity to control your opponent's hand(s), the chance to use a successful leg hooking technique increases.

There are many different types of hooking techniques available in San Shou Kuai Jiao. You can hook an opponent from a standing or kneeling position. Normally, you use the foot or lower leg to hook an opponent's leg or ankle. In many applications, hooking is used as a leg block, and sometimes serves to control a leg attack or to immobilize an opponent.

In many applications, kicking techniques are executed along with hooking techniques. This combination, known as Hook Kicking, is used to lock and uproot your opponent simultaneously. Hook kicks usually target the ankles and lower legs. In general, hook kicks have more power than just a leg hook, so your opponent goes down harder.

But whether hooking or hook kicking, keep in mind that hand techniques are vital to the success of a throw. A hooking technique needs the hands to control an opponent's body. The hand techniques often used along with the hooking techniques are pulling, pushing and thrusting. The hand techniques must have enough power to make the throw effective. Another important element is that the hand(s) and leg(s) must coordinate when executing hooking techniques. Also, the direction of the applied force of the technique must be correct. Generally speaking, the force applied by the hand(s) is in the opposite direction of the hooking leg or foot. This provides maximum symmetry power.

In this chapter we will introduce various types of hooking tech-

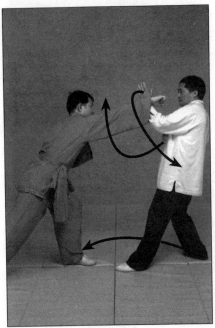

Figure 6-1

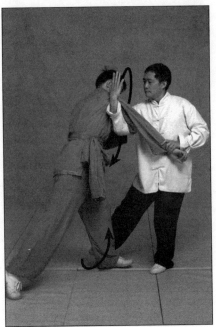

Figure 6-2

niques widely used in fighting. Some of these techniques are suitable for tall and strong people who can take advantage of their longer arms, legs and strength. Examples of these techniques are #2, 8, 9, 10. Other techniques are best suited for smaller and quicker people. Examples of these types of techniques are #4, 6, 7.

6-2. Leg Hooking Techniques

1. Lifting the Elbow, Hooking the Ankle Throw 扛肘摔

a). With his left foot forward, Gray attacks with a right hand punch to White's head. White moves his head to the right to evade the punch and at the same time uses his left hand to block and grab Gray's right wrist (Figure 6-1).

b). In a continuous motion, White thrusts his right forearm under Gray's armpit, bends his elbow and lifts upward. At the same time, White steps forward with his right foot and hooks it behind Gray's left ankle (Figure 6-2).

c). White twists his hip from left to right. Using his left hand, White pulls Gray's right arm down while continuing to lift at the armpit. White simultaneously hooks the left ankle upward. This makes Gray fall backward over White's right leg (Figure 6-3).

Key Points

a). You should pivot to the left on your left foot before you step forward. This will set up a good angle to execute the throw.

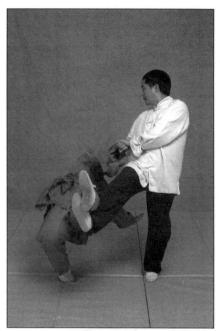

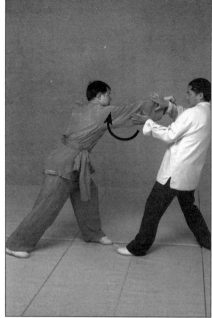

Figure 6-3   Figure 6-4

b). Lifting with your right arm, hooking the foot, and twisting your hips from left to right should happen simultaneously.

c). Throughout the throw, your left leg should be bent for good root and balance.

2. Seizing the Upper Arm, Leg Hooking Throw 拿臂摠摔

a). With his left foot forward, Gray attacks with his right hand. White raises both arms and blocks the punch from left to right. At the same time, White uses his right hand to grab Gray's left wrist or sleeve, and uses his left hand to grab Gray's upper arm (Figure 6-4).

b). White uses both hands to pull Gray's arm downward to the right and hooks the outside of Gray's left ankle with his right foot (Figure 6-5).

c). White continues to pull while lifting Gray's left foot. Gray falls sideways to his left (Figure 6-6).

Key Points

a). Pivot to the left on your left foot before you step forward. This will set up a good angle to execute the throw.

b). During the throw, push and press on your opponent's right arm to your right.

c). Your left foot should be bent to keep good root and balance throughout the technique.

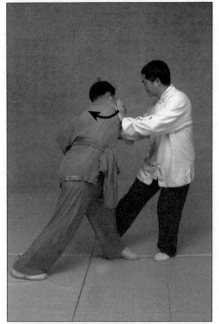

Figure 6-5

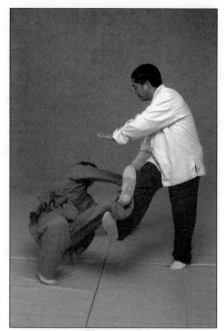

Figure 6-6

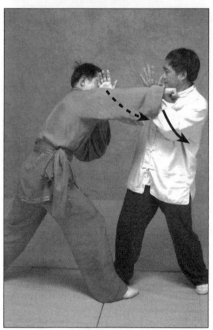

Figure 6-7

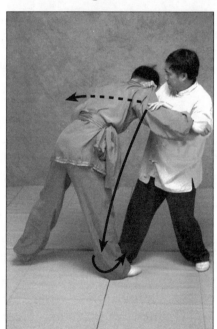

Figure 6-8

3. **Picking Up the Leg Throw** 撿腿摔(勾)

a). With his right foot forward, Gray attacks with a right punch to the head. White blocks the punch with both hands and follows by grabbing Gray's shirt at the chest or right shoulder and pulling him forward (Figures 6-7 and 6-8).

b). Gray resists and tries to pull backward. While Gray struggles, White slips his right foot forward and behind Gray's right ankle, lifts his foot up, and catches it with his left hand (Figure 6-9).

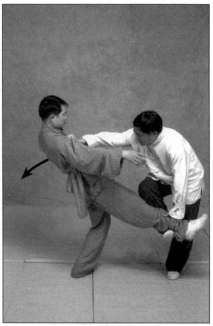

Figure 6-9

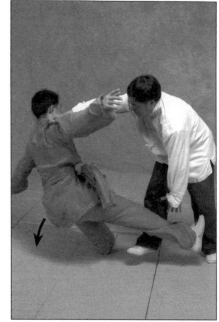

Figure 6-10

c). As White lifts Gray's right leg, he pushes Gray's chest with his right hand to make Gray fall backward (Figure 6-10).

Key Points

a). Keep your left leg bent for good rooting.

b). All the movements must be done quickly and continuously so your opponent has no chance to stabilize himself.

c). The final push must be forceful and strong.

4. Hooking the Leg Throw 勾帶腳

a). With his left foot forward Gray attacks with a right punch. White blocks with his left hand and slides his right foot behind Gray's left ankle. White's right hand is free to strike Gray in the face or block an attack (Figure 6-11).

b). White steps backward with his left foot while pulling Gray's right arm down and forward. Simultaneously, White hooks Gray's right foot and drags it forward to take him down (Figures 6-12, 6-13 and 6-14).

Key Points

a). Step backward as far as possible to create more distance to drag the leg.

b). When hooking and dragging your opponent's foot, your other leg must be bent for good root and balance.

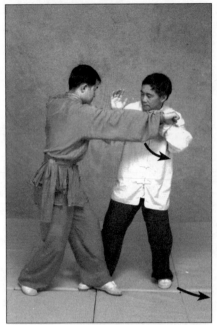

Figure 6-11

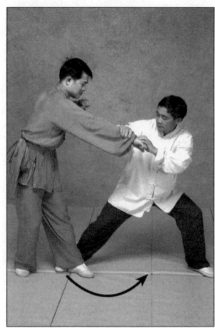

Figure 6-12

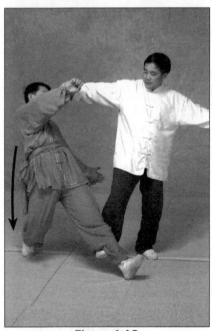

Figure 6-13

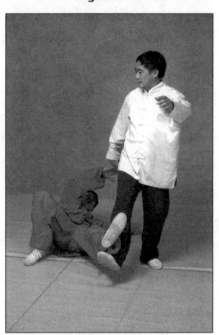

Figure 6-14

5. **Hook Kicking, Leg Sweeping Throw** 勾踢殺腳腿

a). With his right foot forward, Gray attacks with his right hand. White moves his head slightly to the left and blocks with his right hand, and extends his left hand to shield then grab Gray's right elbow. Simultaneously, White executes a right hook kick to Gray's right lower leg (Figure 6-15).

b). Gray detects the kick and lifts his right leg to avoid it (Figure 6-16).

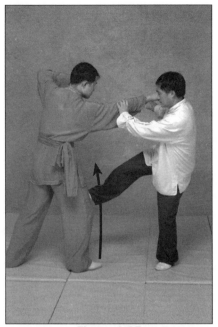

Figure 6-15

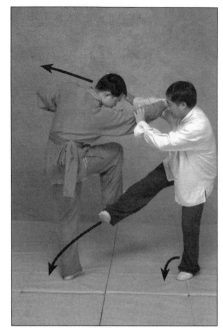

Figure 6-16

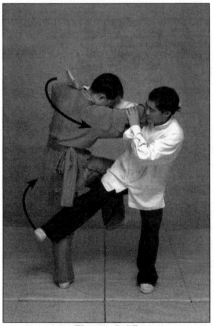

Figure 6-17

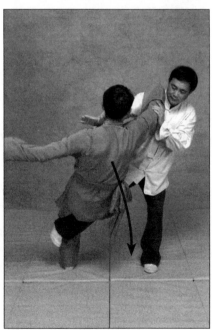

Figure 6-18

c). White pivots to the left on the ball of his left foot and extends his right foot to the back of Gray's left leg (Figures 6-17).

d). Continuing the above movement, White twists counter-clockwise and uses his right leg to sweep Gray's supporting leg. Simultaneously, White strikes Gray with his right arm across the upper body to make him fall (Figure 6-18).

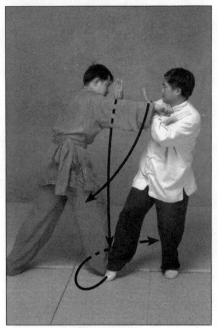

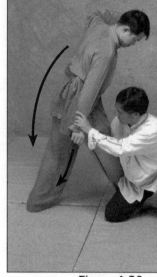

Figure 6-19   **Figure 6-20**

Key Points

a). For good balance, keep your left knee bent when pivoting to the left.

b). The sweep must be powerful and coordinated with the upper body.

6. Lower Inner Hooking Throw 小得合

a). With his right foot forward, Gray attacks with his right hand. White blocks the punch with his left hand then grabs the wrist. At the same time, White strikes Gray in the arm or face with his right hand (Figure 6-19).

b). Next, White curls his right leg outside and around Gray's right foot while lowering himself to the ground to hook Gray at the ankle. White keeps his right knee touching the ground in a kneeling position, and controls Gray's right arm by pulling it downward (Figure 6-20).

c). White uses his right lower leg to pinch Gray's ankle, and then strikes Gray's thigh with an elbow or shoulder to make Gray fall on his back (Figures 6-21 and 6-22).

Key Points

a). After hooking your opponent's leg, you must squat down and strike his leg as quickly as possible.

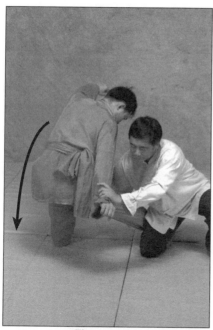

Figure 6-21

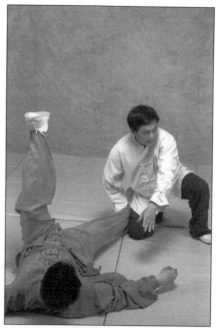

Figure 6-22

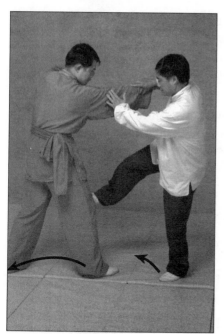

Figure 6-23

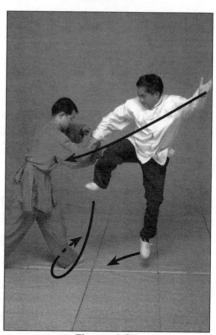

Figure 6-24

7. Hook Kicking, Lower Inner Hooking Throw 勾踢小得合

a). With his right foot forward, Gray attacks with his right hand. White blocks his attack with both hands, from left to right. Simultaneously, White executes a hook kick to Gray's right lower leg with his right foot (Figure 6-23).

b). If Gray withdraws his right foot to evade the kick and steps back, White hops one step forward with his left leg (Figure 6-24).

111

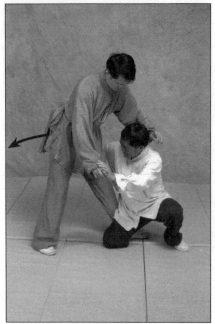

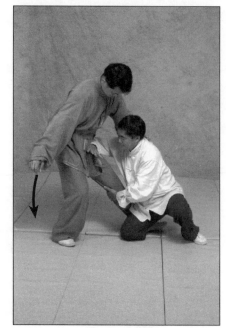

| Figure 6-25 | Figure 6-26 |

c). White then squats on his left leg, hooks his right leg around Gray's lower left leg, and squeezes. White's right knee touches the ground in a kneeling position. With his left hand White pulls Gray's right arm downward to control its movement (Figure 6-25).

d). White then grabs Gray's left leg with his left hand and uses his right elbow to strike and press downward on Gray's upper thigh to make him fall on his back (Figures 6-26 and 6-27).

Key Points

a). After hooking your opponent's leg, you must quickly strike and knock him over.

b). Another variation of this technique is that your opponent only lifts his leg out of the way instead of moving back. You also can apply technique # 5 to throw him.

8. Pulling the Neck, Hook Kicking Throw 拔頸勾踢

a). With his right foot forward, Gray attacks with his right hand. White blocks to the left with the left hand and grabs Gray's forearm or wrist (Figure 6-28).

b). White extends his right hand past Gray's right shoulder and hooks the back of his neck. White pulls Gray's head back and downward to the right. Simultaneously, White uses his right leg to execute the hook kick to Gray's front leg to make him fall (Figures 6-29 and 6-30).

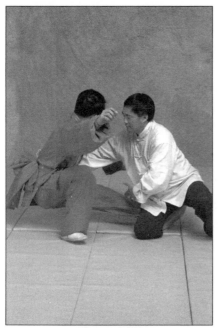

Figure 6-27

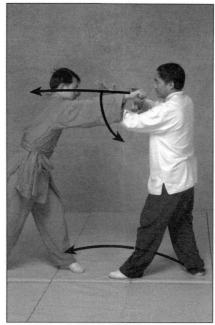

Figure 6-28

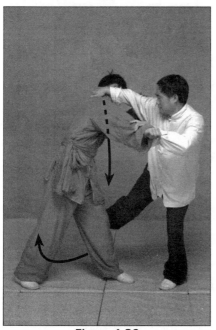

Figure 6-29

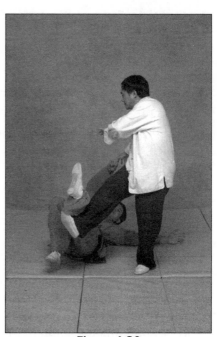

Figure 6-30

Key Points

a). Your supporting left leg should stay bent when executing the technique.

b). Before you kick, make sure your opponent's body is off balance and leaning forward to his left, with most of his body weight on the front leg.

c). Kick and pull simultaneously.

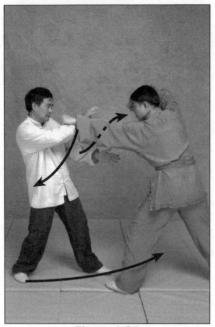

Figure 6-31

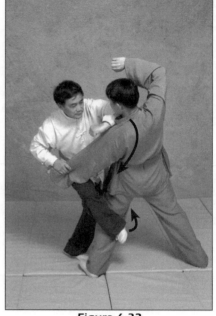

Figure 6-32

9. Outside Suspending the Leg Hooking Throw 外勾挂

a). With his left foot forward, Gray attacks with his left hand. White blocks to the right with his right hand and grabs Gray's forearm. White slips his left foot forward and places it in front of Gray's left foot to close the distance (Figure 6-31).

b). White then uses his right foot to hook the hollow of Gray's left knee. At the same time, White strikes with his left elbow and presses forward against the neck or chest. His right hand keeps pulling Gray to the rear (Figure 6-32).

c). As Gray loses his balance, White continues to hook Gray's left leg up and towards him. White pulls and presses and then turns his body quickly to the right to topple Gray (Figure 6-33).

Key Points

a). The pulling, pressing and hooking movements must happen simultaneously.

b). Keep your left knee bent for good balance.

10. Pulling, Hook Kicking Throw 扯拉勾踢

a). With his left foot forward, Gray attacks with his left hand. White blocks the attack with his left hand, grabs the wrist, and uses his right hand to strike Gray's upper arm (Figure 6-34).

b). White then jerks Gray's arm down and uses his right hand to

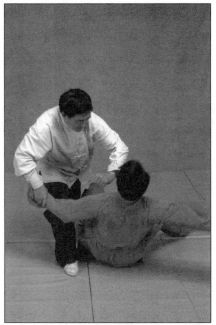

Figure 6-33

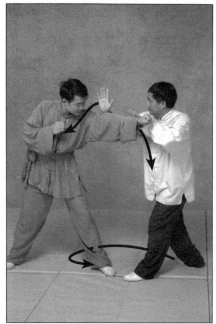

Figure 6-34

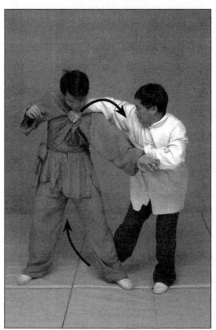

Figure 6-35

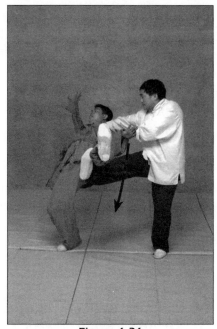

Figure 6-36

grab Gray's shirt. Simultaneously, he steps in with his right leg and hooks Gray's left leg upward (Figure 6-35).

c). White pulls Gray backward while hooking up and to the left to make Gray fall on his back (Figure 6-36).

Key Points

a). Block to the outside when your opponent strikes at you.

b). The pull and the hook kick must be strong and simultaneous.

115

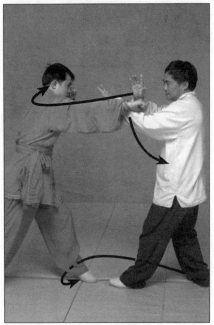

Figure 6-37

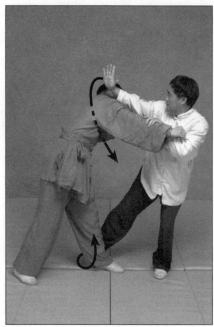

Figure 6-38

11. Chopping, Hook Kicking Throw 劈掌勾踢

a). With his left foot forward, Gray attacks with his right hand. White blocks with his left hand and then grabs Gray's wrist (Figure 6-37).

b). With his left foot, White pivots slightly to the left for better balance and pulls Gray closer. White then chops with his right hand to the right side of Gray's neck while using his right foot to kick and hook Gray's left leg. Gray's body weight is on his left foot and leaning forward (Figure 6-38).

c). White's chopping hand presses downward to the right while his leg hooks upward to knock Gray on his back (Figure 6-39).

Key Points

a). When kicking, keep your supporting leg slightly bent for good balance.

12. Holding the Leg, Chopping the Neck and Hook Kicking Throw 摟腿劈掌勾踢

a). Gray throws a right roundhouse kick to White's left. White uses the **Palm and Elbow Crossing Method** (left arm slightly bent with the elbow pointing out, the right palm facing outward and leaning against the left upper arm) to intercept his kick (Figure 6-40).

b). White then scoops his left hand outward and upward to catch Gray's leg and destroy his balance. White extends his right leg to kick and hook Gray's left foot, and chops Gray's neck with his right palm (Figure 6-41).

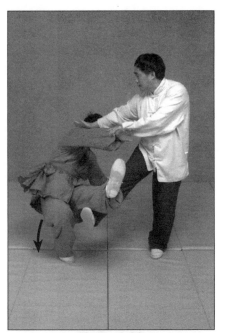

Figure 6-39

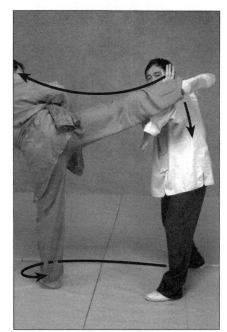

Figure 6-40

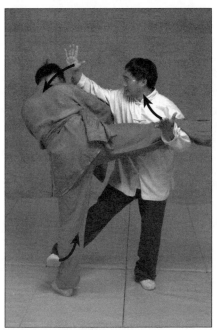

Figure 6-41

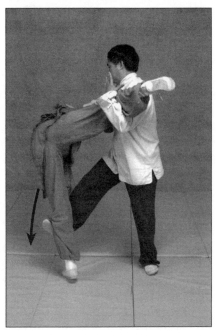

Figure 6-42

c). White continues to lift Gray's leg, and then presses forward, using the hook to keep Gray from moving his leg. Gray then topples to the side (Figure 6-42).

Key Points

a). After catching your opponent's kicking leg, step forward with your left foot to get the correct distance for the throw.

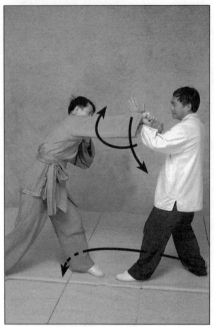

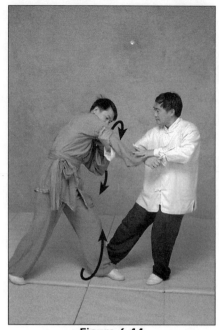

| Figure 6-43 | Figure 6-44 |

b). Lift the kicking leg as high as you can to keep your opponent off balance.

13. Lifting the Elbow, Hooking Sideways Throw 扛肘勾踢

a). With his left foot forward, Gray attacks with his right hand. White moves his head to the right to avoid the punch. At the same time he blocks with the left hand and grabs Gray's wrist (Figure 6-43).

b). White pulls Gray's right arm down and pivots his left foot to the left. Then White uses his right arm to scoop under Gray's right armpit. Simultaneously he kicks and hooks Gray's left ankle with his right (Figure 6-44).

c). White hooks the leg upward and lifts Gray up and to the right. Simultaneously, White twists to the right to uproot and throw Gray to the ground (Figure 6-45).

Key Points

a). Make sure you have the right distance so you can hook your opponent's front leg.

b). Throughout the technique, keep your left foot well bent for good root and balance.

14. Suspending the Leg Hook, Striking the Back Throw
勾掛砸背

a). Gray attacks with a right hook to the head. White quickly

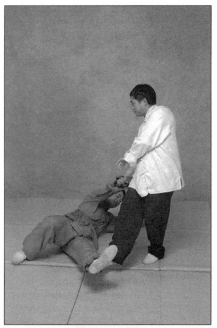

Figure 6-45

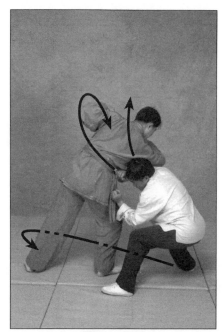

Figure 6-46

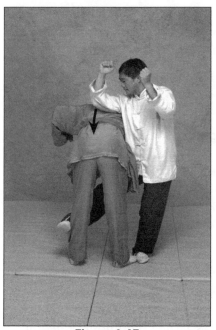

Figure 6-47

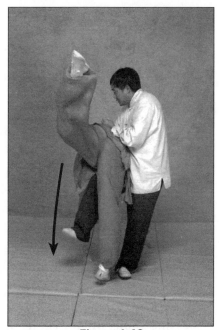

Figure 6-48

squats down to evade the attack, his left foot forward and to the right of Gray (Figure 6-46).

b). White then springs up on Gray's right side and extends his right leg to hook and lock Gray's left leg. Simultaneously, White strikes Gray's back with an elbow (or both arms) and turns his body to the right to take Gray down (Figures 6-47 and 6-48).

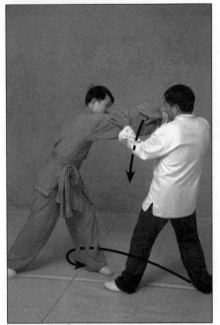

Figure 6-49

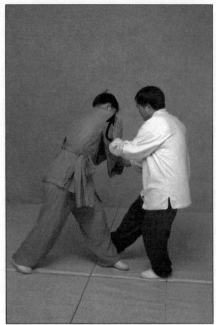

Figure 6-50

Key Points

a). When squatting down to evade your opponent's attack, keep your head low and always watch your opponent.

b). You should spring up immediately after you dodge the right hook.

15. Suspending Leg Hook, Pushing the Shoulder Throw 勾挂擠靠

a). With his left foot forward, Gray attacks with a right punch to the head. White leans back slightly to dodge the attack. At the same time he blocks from left to right with both hands and grabs Gray's right arm (Figure 6-49).

b). White extends his right leg to hook Gray's left ankle and uses his right hand to pull Gray downward (Figure 6-50).

c). White slides his left hand forward to Gray's right shoulder. Simultaneously, he hooks Gray's left foot up to the left, twists his body to the right, and pushes Gray's shoulder, causing Gray to fall to the left (Figure 6-51).

Key Points

a). Keep your left leg bent throughout the throw.

b). You can step forward with your left foot to set up the correct distance for the throw.

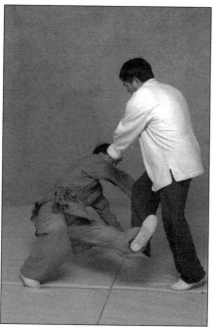

Figure 6-51

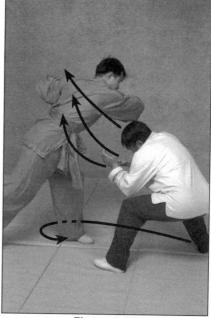

Figure 6-52

16. Dodging, Hooking the Leg, and Pushing Throw
閃身勾挂擠靠

a). Gray attacks with a right lateral hook to the head. White squats down quickly to evade the attack, his left foot stepping forward to get close and to the right of Gray (Figure 6-52).

b). White extends his right leg behind Gray's left ankle to hook the ankle and prevent Gray from moving his foot away. Simultaneously, White springs up and uses both hands to strike Gray. White uses both hands and also his body to press and push Gray and knock him to the ground (Figures 6-53 and 6-54).

Key Points

a). When squatting down to dodge the attack, keep your head low and always watch your opponent.

b). When pushing your opponent, root your rear foot to the ground and drive forward from the back leg. This will create more power for the push.

17. Hooking the Front and Sweeping the Back Throw
前勾后掃

a). Gray is in a fighting stance with his left foot forward. White initiates the attack by faking a right punch, and immediately follows the fake by executing a right hook kick at Gray's left ankle. Gray lifts his foot or steps back to evade White's attack (Figure 6-55).

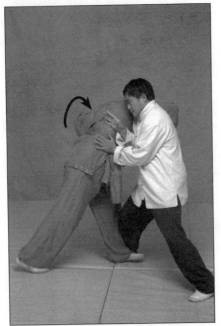

Figure 6-53

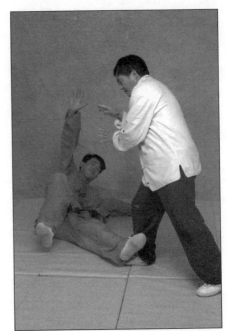

Figure 6-54

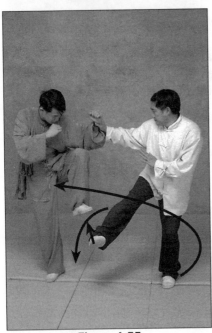

Figure 6-55

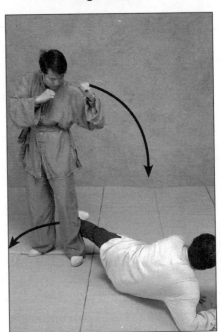

Figure 6-56

b). White drops to the floor, squatting on his right leg and supporting his body with both hands. White then spins his body
to the left and uses his left leg to sweep Gray's ankle or lower
leg to make him fall backward (Figures 6-56 and 6-57).

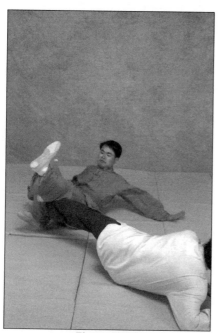

Figure 6-57

Key Points

a). In order to sweep your opponent successfully, you must make full use of the body's spinning momentum by sweeping through your opponent's leg or legs.

b). Avoid your opponent landing on your legs when he falls.

Chapter 7
Other Throwing Methods

其他摔法

7-1. Introduction

In the previous three chapters, we introduced San Shou Kuai Jiao techniques that have similar characteristics and we grouped them together to make them easy to remember. You can choose and specialize in techniques from this book that most fit your body type and fighting style. However, having a broad knowledge of many different types of techniques is also very important, and will give you an advantage in a fight. Techniques used in fighting should be diverse, alive, and spontaneous. If a technique that you apply to an opponent is not working, you should automatically use a second technique, then a third, and so on until your opponent is thrown. Generally speaking, the more techniques you can use in a fight, the more ammunition you have. Your opponent will have a harder time discerning what move you are going to make next.

However, if you know hundreds of techniques but have mastered none of them, they are useless and you have wasted your time and energy. It is better to master a few techniques first, and then add more as you gain in experience and improve your skills.

There are many different throwing methods for taking down an opponent. It is impossible to learn and master them all. It is also hard to say which technique is best. The same technique can be applied differently by different people because of varying body types and strength. But no matter what method you use, an effective technique needs to be skillful, alive, fast and powerful. In fighting, you can not plan what techniques you will use against your opponent. You need to respond naturally to what your opponent does, and counter with appropriate techniques.

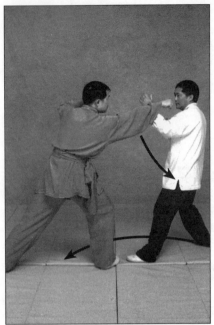

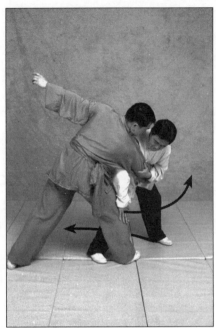

| Figure 7-1 | Figure 7-2 |

In this chapter, we will introduce techniques often used in San Shou fighting. Each one has its own characteristics and different applications. When practicing, avoid using brute force. This will help you to develop techniques that rely on good skills instead of just strength. Keep thinking and analyzing every technique so you can make each one work better for you. You are encouraged to use techniques that you learn here as a foundation to create your own.

7-2. Throwing Techniques

1. Hand Blocking, Sideways Throw 手別側摔

a). With his right foot forward, Gray attacks with his right hand. White uses his left hand to block the punch (Figure 7-1).

b). White grabs and locks Gray's right arm under his left armpit while stepping forward and placing his right foot between Gray's legs. With his right hand White presses Gray's knee to upset his balance. White also uses his right shoulder to press tightly against Gray's right upper arm (Figure 7-2).

c). Simultaneously, White steps his left foot back and behind the right leg so that his back is to Gray. In a continuous motion, White turns quickly to the left as far as possible while pulling Gray's right arm and pressing the knee. This causes Gray to spin and hit the ground (Figure 7-3).

Key Points

a). You must break your opponent's balance first by placing your

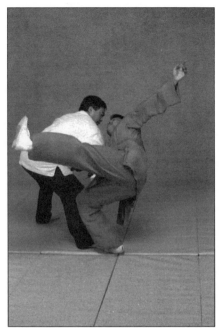

Figure 7-3

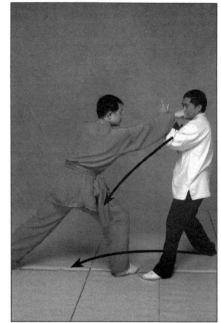

Figure 7-4

right hand on the side of his right knee and pressing firmly down.

b). Keep your hip pressed against your opponent's lower abdomen throughout the throw.

c). Use the turning momentum of your body to throw your opponent.

d). You must pull the arm, push the knee and turn the body in a smooth, powerful motion.

2. **Hand Blocking, Moving Forward Throw** 手別前進摔

a). With his right foot forward, Gray attacks with his right hand. White blocks the punch with his left forearm and locks Gray's arm under his armpit, or grabs Gray's upper sleeve (Figure 7-4).

b). With his right hand, White reaches for the outside of Gray's right leg and presses firmly on the hollow of his knee. Still pressing, White steps quickly forward with his right foot as if speeding past Gray's right leg. Simultaneously, White uses his right shoulder to strike and press against Gray's upper arm, knocking Gray backwards (Figure 7-5).

Key Points

a). Keep your opponent off balance throughout the throw by pressing firmly on the hollow of his right knee.

b). When stepping forward, both knees should be well bent for good balance.

127

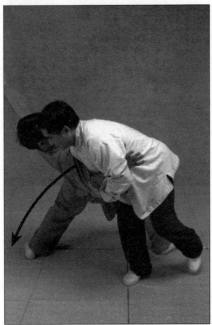

Figure 7-5

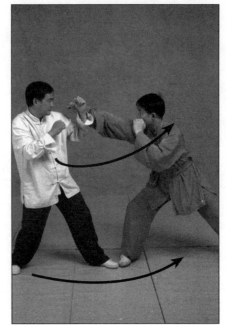

Figure 7-6

3. Crossing Elbow Strike, Pressing the Neck Throw

橫肘頂摔

a). With his right foot forward, Gray attacks with a right hand to the head. White uses his left hand to block the punch (Figure 7-6).

b). White steps forward with his right foot and places it deep between Gray's legs. White locks Gray's right arm under his left armpit, hits Gray with a right elbow to the face or neck, and continues to press forward and to the left with his right elbow (Figures 7-7).

c). White then steps his left foot behind and around his right foot. White pulls Gray's right arm down and backward to the left and continues to move quickly to the left to make Gray fall backward (Figure 7-8).

Key Points

a). The stepping has to be quick and smooth in order to gain momentum for the throw.

b). When applying the throw, your left arm should continue to pull your opponent's right arm to your left. Your right arm must also keep pressing your opponent's neck downward to the left to keep him off balance throughout the throw.

4. Moving Forward, Cutting the Neck Throw 上步切摔

a). With his right foot forward, Gray attacks with a right hand to the face. White leans slightly backward to evade the attack

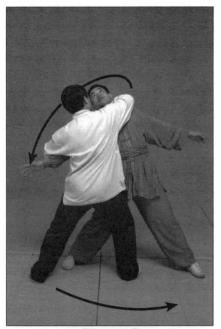

Figure 7-7

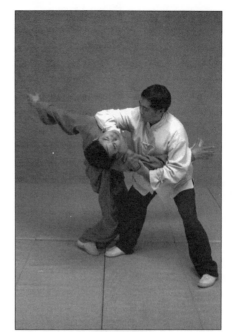

Figure 7-8

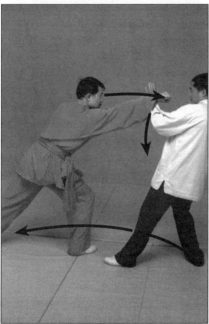

Figure 7-9

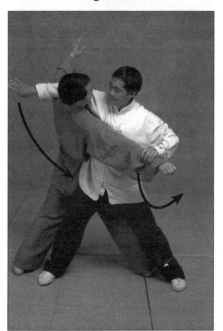

Figure 7-10

and at the same time uses his left arm to block the punch from left to right (Figure 7-9).

b). Following the above motion, White grabs Gray's right wrist or sleeve and steps forward and behind Gray's right leg. Using the thumb side of his right palm or the inner side of his forearm, White slashes Gray's throat and then hooks his neck (Figure 7-10).

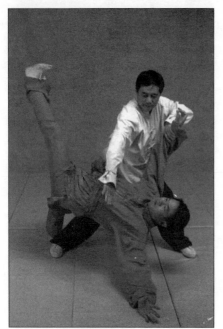

Figure 7-11

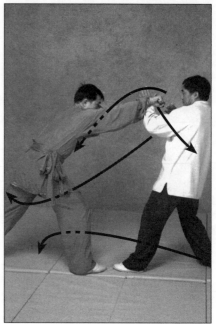

Figure 7-12

c). White continues to push Gray's right arm outward and down, then twists to the left and presses his right arm against Gray's neck while pressing his right hip against Gray's waist to throw him down (Figure 7-11).

Key Points

a). The forward step has to be quick. Put your opponent immediately off balance by pressing forward with your body and getting your right hip against his waist.

b). Your left hand should pull your opponent's right arm throughout the throw.

c). For maximum power, twist your body from right to left and keep good root and balance.

5. Scooping the Groin, Crossing Back Throw 挑襠過背摔

a). Gray attacks with a right punch to the head. White blocks it with his left arm and grabs Gray at the forearm (Figure 7-12).

b). Simultaneously, White steps forward and puts his right foot between Gray's legs and squats down. White thrusts his right arm between Gray's legs and scoops upward while pressing his shoulder into Gray's lower abdomen. With his left hand White keeps pulling Gray's right arm down to the left (Figure 7-13).

c). White then springs up, straightening his body and lifting Gray off the ground. White continues the scooping motion with his

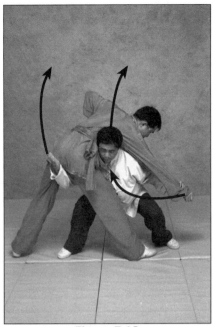

Figure 7-13

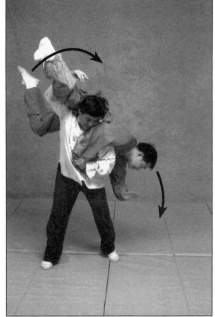

Figure 7-14

right arm to get Gray onto his shoulder, then pulls Gray's right arm downward and to the left to throw him to the ground (Figure 7-14).

Key Points

a.) You must get your opponent off balance before getting underneath him.

b.) Lift quickly. Do not give your opponent time to use his weight against you.

6. Stomach Throw 倒地拉臂蹬腹過頂摔

a). Gray seizes White by the neck or the upper arms. White grabs Gray's sleeves or shoulders with both arms and pulls him down and forward (Figure 7-15).

b). At the same time, White drops his body straight to the ground on his buttocks to make Gray lean forward. Both hands keep pulling Gray down. As Gray falls forward, White puts his right foot against Gray's abdomen, then rolls backward from the buttocks to the back (Figure 7-16).

c). As he pulls with both hands, White straightens his right leg to flip Gray over his head (Figure 7-17).

Key Points

a). When dropping your body, go straight to the ground on your buttocks.

b). Both hands must pull throughout the throw.

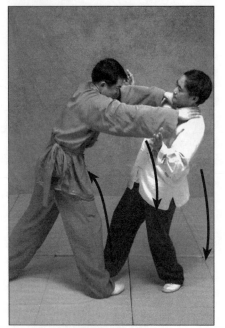

Figure 7-15

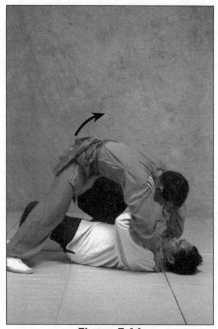

Figure 7-16

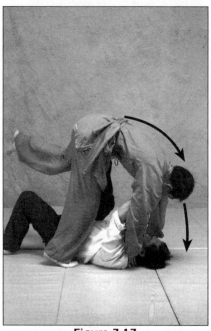

Figure 7-17

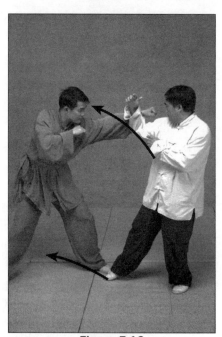

Figure 7-18

7. Pulling the Leg, Pressing Forward Throw 拉腳前推

a). With his left foot forward, Gray attacks with a left hand strike to the head. White blocks the strike with his right arm. (Figure 7-18).

b). White counters with a left hand strike to Gray's face and steps his right foot deep between Gray's legs (Figure 7-19).

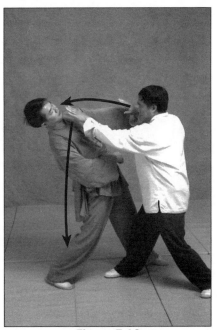

Figure 7-19

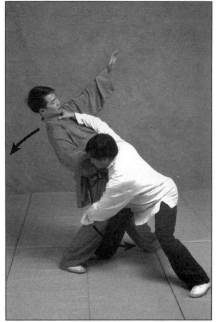

Figure 7-20

c). As Gray attempts to block the strike, White drops his body and slips his left hand down and behind Gray's right knee. White holds the knee tightly and pulls it back and upward. At the same time, White slides his right hand forward and under Gray's chin and pushes forward and down, forcing Gray to topple over backwards (Figure 7-20).

Key Points

a). Step deep between your opponent's legs to reach his back knee.

b). Pull the knee and push the chin or neck simultaneously to create symmetry power.

8. Dodging, Scooping the Groin, Pressing the Neck Throw 閃身掏襠按頸

a). Gray attacks with a right hook to the head. White squats down to evade the punch. Simultaneously, he slides his right foot forward to Gray's right and strikes Gray in the ribs with his right elbow. (Figure 7-21).

b). Without stopping, White steps his left foot forward. Before Gray can turn his body and strike back, White springs up and uses his right forearm to strike downward to Gray's neck, then encircles his neck and presses downward. Simultaneously, White uses his left hand to scoop Gray's groin from behind (Figure 7-22a and 7-22b).

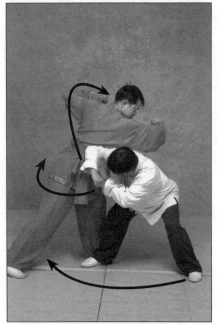

Figure 7-21

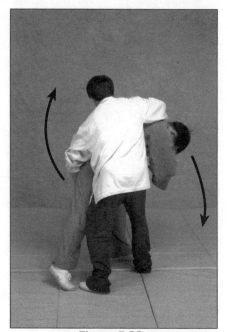

Figure 7-22a

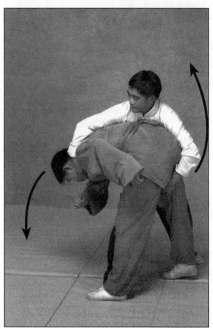

Figure 7-22b

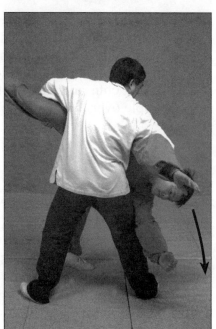

Figure 7-23

c). Simultaneously scooping the groin upward and pressing the neck downward to his right, White tosses Gray headfirst to the ground (Figure 7-23).

Key Points

a). Keep your body low when dodging and slide to the outside of your opponent's punching hand. Once you are in, keep close to his body to give him less room to hit you.

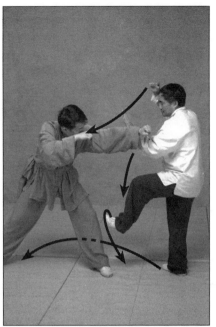

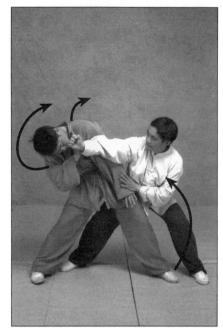

| Figure 7-24 | Figure 7-25 |

b). When you scoop upward with the left hand, you can grab your opponent's pants or his leg.

9. Controlling the Leg and Pushing the Chest Throw

躍步管腳攔胸

a). With his left foot forward, Gray attacks with a left hand punch. White leans back slightly to dodge the attack and uses his left hand to slap the punch downward. At the same time, White picks up his left foot (Figure 7-24).

b). White steps down and slides his right foot forward and places it behind Gray's right foot. White uses his left hand to seal Gray's left hand and at the same time punches Gray in the face with his right hand (Figure 7-25).

c). White then twists to the right with his right arm pressing against Gray's chest. White can also strike Gray's neck or head. Finally, White pushes Gray over his right leg, throwing him to the ground (Figure 7-26).

Key Points

a). When applying the throw, use your right knee to press and jerk against the back of your opponent's front leg to uproot him.

b). The leg lift in the first move can be used to stomp on your opponent's foot. After stepping down or stomping, keep your body low.

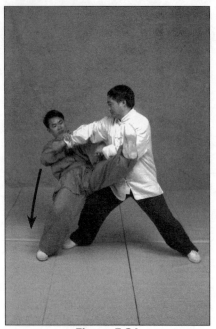

Figure 7-26

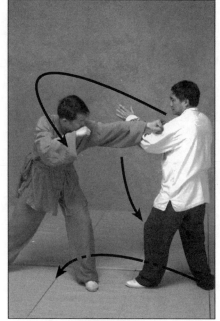

Figure 7-27

10. Surrounding the Neck, Pulling Backward Throw

圈頸后拉

a). With his left foot forward, Gray attacks with a left hand strike. White blocks it with his left hand from left to right (Figure 7-27).

b). White grabs Gray's left arm, steps forward around him and puts his right foot behind Gray's feet. Once around, White pushes Gray's left hand down and uses his right hand to wrap Gray in a headlock or neck lock (Figure 7-28).

c). White then steps out to the left with his left foot, both hands still controlling Gray. White squeezes Gray's neck and pulls downward to his left (Figure 7-29).

d). Using his right hip as a turning point, White turns quickly to the left to throw Gray down (Figure 7-30).

Key Points

a). Intercepting the attack, stepping forward, and wrapping your opponent in the headlock should happen simultaneously.

b). Your supporting leg should be bent to keep good balance so that when you execute the throw you do not fall with your opponent.

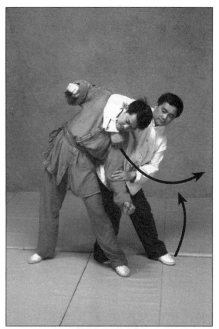

Figure 7-28

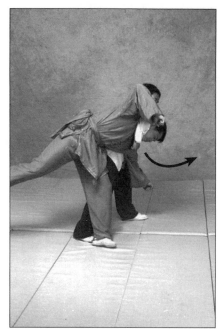

Figure 7-29

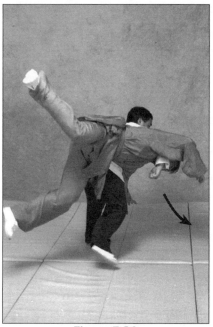

Figure 7-30

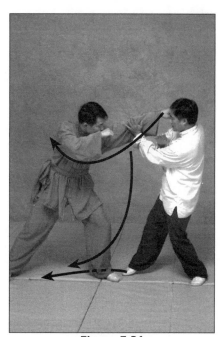

Figure 7-31

11. Flipping Over Throw 提翻

a). Gray attacks with his left hand with his left foot forward. White leans back slightly to dodge the attack and blocks with his left hand (Figure 7-31).

b). White steps in quickly with the right foot and places it behind Gray's legs. Simultaneously, he grabs Gray's chest or shoulder and uses his right forearm to press backward and slips his left

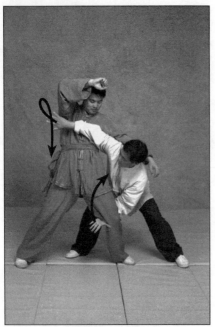

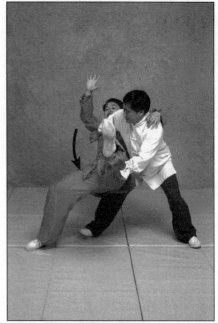

| Figure 7-32 | Figure 7-33 |

hand behind Gray's left leg (Figure 7-32).

c). White turns to the right with his right arm pressing Gray's chest while his left hand scoops upward to throw Gray to the floor (Figure 7-33).

Key Points

a). Step in deep so that your front leg is behind your opponent's front leg and your body is low. Press your opponent's chest to make him lose his balance before the throw.

b). When executing the throw, apply force in opposite directions to create strong symmetry power.

12. Brushing the Neck, Blocking the Knee Throw

抹脖攔膝摔

a). Gray attacks with his right hand. White leans backward slightly to dodge the attack. At the same time he uses his right hand to block the punch to the right, White strikes with his left hand and seals Gray's right elbow (Figures 7-34 and 7-35).

b). White then moves forward quickly and with his right hand grabs the back of Gray's neck and presses downward (Figure 7-36).

c). Simultaneously, his left hand moves downward to block Gray's knee and limit his leg movement (Figure 7-37).

d). White steps back to the right with his right foot. Simultaneously, he presses down on Gray's neck and scoops Gray's knee to throw him to the ground (Figures 7-38 and 7-39).

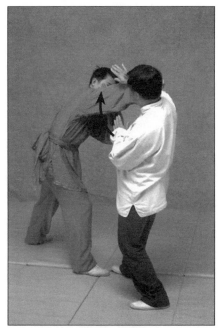

Figure 7-34

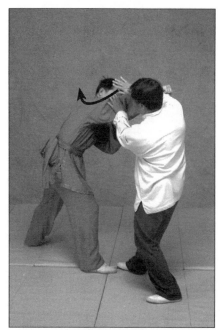

Figure 7-35

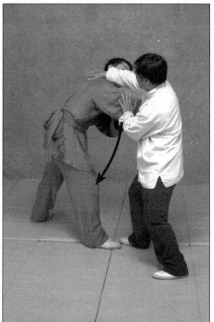

Figure 7-36

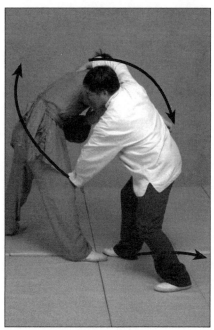

Figure 7-37

Key Points

a). Both hands need to coordinate to create symmetry power for the throw.

13. Twisting the Neck Throw 搓頸摔

a). Gray locks White in a bear hug. White uses both hands to hold Gray's head and twist it sideways and downward (Figure 7-40).

139

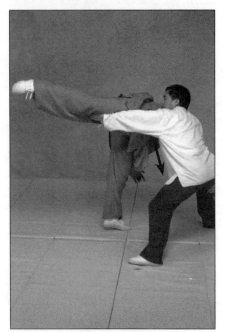

Figure 7-38

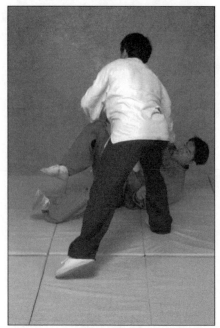

Figure 7-39

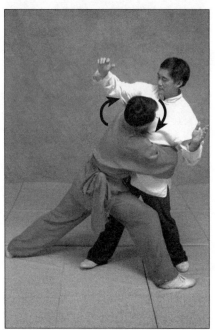

Figure 7-40

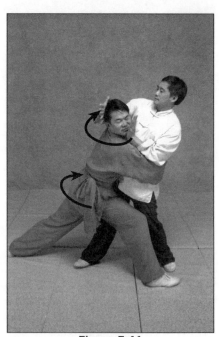

Figure 7-41

b). Simultaneously White turns his body in the direction of the head twist to throw Gray to the ground (Figures 7-41 and 7-42).

Key Points
a). You can step back with your front foot to avoid the bear hug and create more room for your body to turn.

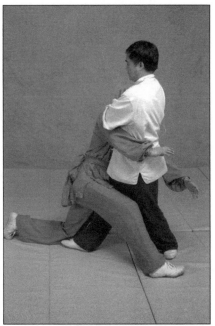

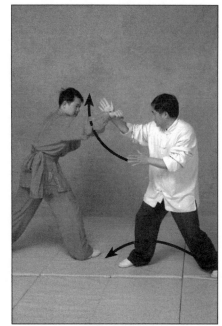

| Figure 7-42 | Figure 7-43 |

b). When practicing with a partner, be very careful not to twist the head with power and inadvertently break your partner's neck.

14. Sweeping the Leg Throw 殺腳腿

a). Gray attacks with his right hand with his right foot forward. White blocks the punch with his right hand from right to left (Figure 7-43).

b). Then White switches hands and grabs Gray's forearm with his left hand. Simultaneously, White crosses his left foot behind his right (also called **Steal Foot Step**, because it is concealed from your opponent) and places it in front of Gray's right foot. White reaches his right arm around the left side of Gray's head (Figure 7-44).

c). Without stopping, White sweeps Gray's right lower leg from left to right and to the back. Simultaneously, White strikes the side of Gray's head or neck with a crossing chop. White continues to pull Gray's left arm downward to the left to make Gray fall on his back (Figures 7-45 and 7-46).

Key Points

a). When cross-stepping to close the distance between you and your opponent, move as quickly as possible to give your opponent no chance to detect your intention.

b). Both knees should be bent, and keep your supporting leg bent when executing the throw.

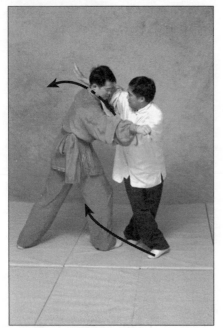

Figure 7-44

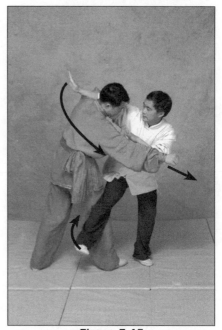

Figure 7-45

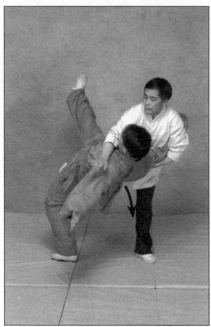

Figure 7-46

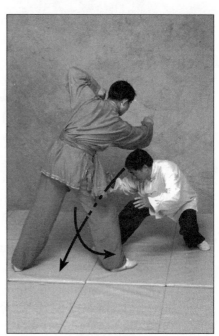

Figure 7-47

    c). Coordinate the hand strike and leg sweep for symmetry power.

15. Penetrating the Legs, Pressing and Rolling Sideways Throw 鑽襠滾壓

    a). Gray attacks with a right hand strike. White ducks to evade the attack and leaps forward between Gray's legs (Figures 7-47 and 7-48).

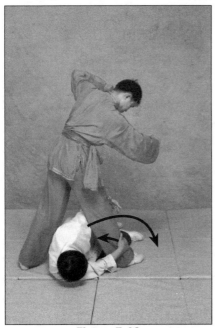

Figure 7-48

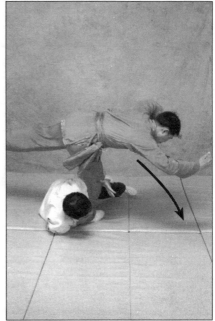

Figure 7-49

b). White uses both hands to hold Gray's right leg (or left leg) tightly and pull it into his chest. White rolls to the right (or to the left) to take Gray down (Figure 7-49).

Key Points

a). After taking your opponent to the ground, you can roll on top of him and follow up with an elbow strike.

16. Leaping and Pushing Forward Throw 虎扑前推

a). Gray reaches for White's neck or shoulders (Figure 7-50).

b). White uses both hands to block Gray's hands upward from the inside and leaps forward to put his front foot between Gray's legs (Figures 7-51 and 7-52).

c). Simultaneously, White pushes from his back foot to generate greater power and uses both palms to strike and push Gray's chest. The shoulders or neck are also appropriate targets (Figure 7-53).

Key Points

a). When leaping forward, your front foot should pass your opponent's center line to gain more control of your opponent's balance and create more compression force before the push.

b). When pushing forward, think of pushing *through* your opponent.

c). Generate the pushing power from the rear leg.

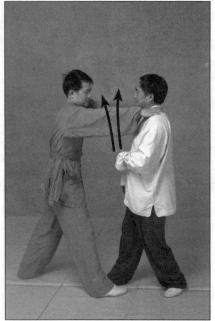

Figure 7-50

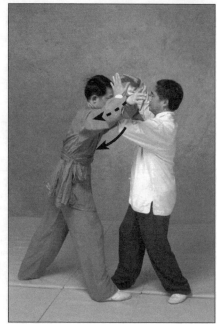

Figure 7-51

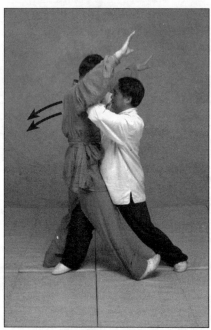

Figure 7-52

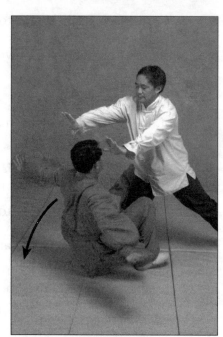

Figure 7-53

17. Penetrating the Legs, Leaning Against the Body Throw 穿腿靠

a). With his left foot forward, Gray attacks with his right hand. (White may also initiate the attack.) White uses his left hand to block from right to left and grabs Gray's right hand (Figure 7-54).

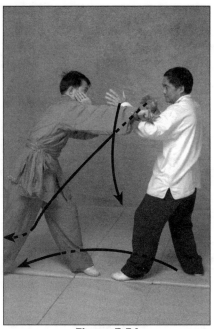

Figure 7-54

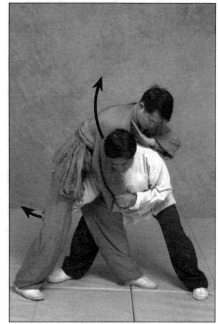

Figure 7-55

b). White pulls Gray's right arm downward and steps his right foot forward behind Gray's left leg to block his left leg. At the same time White sinks downward and slips his right arm between Gray's legs to hook the hollow of his right knee. White continues to pull Gray's right arm (Figure 7-55).

c). White leans forward and uses his right shoulder to strike and press against Gray's chest. White turns his body to the right and uses his right knee to press Gray's left leg from behind and upward simultaneously. He scoops Gray's right leg at the same time to throw him backward and down (Figures 7-56 and 7-57).

Key Points

a). When you step behind your opponent's left leg, squat low for good root and balance.

b). Pull your opponent's right arm downward throughout the technique to prevent him from attacking you.

c). Press your upper body against your opponent's body to uproot him, then execute the throw.

18. Falling Sideways, Pushing the Shoulder Throw 側倒推肩

a). With his left foot forward, Gray attacks with a right hand punch. White blocks it with his left hand from right to left and grabs Gray's forearm (Figure 7-58).

b). White steps his right foot forward and places it inside Gray's left foot while pulling Gray's right arm close in to his chest. At

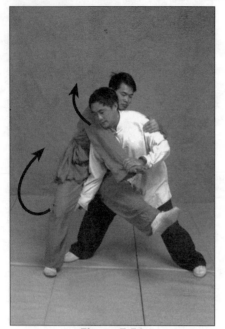

Figure 7-56

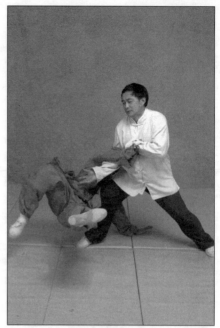

Figure 7-57

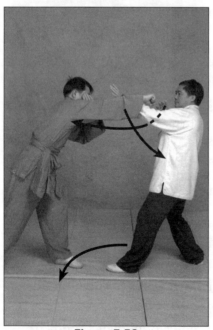

Figure 7-58

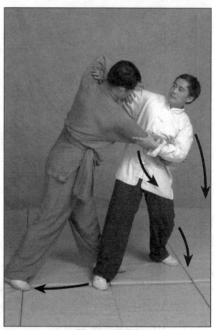

Figure 7-59

this point, Gray's balance is forward and slightly twisted to the right. White can use his right hand to strike Gray in the face or control Gray's right hand (Figure 7-59).

c). White then drops his body sideways and slides his right leg forward, using his right leg to block Gray's foot. White continues to fall sideways onto the ground and to his left (Figure 7-60).

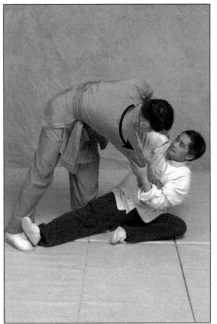

Figure 7-60

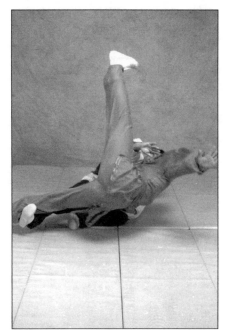

Figure 7-61

d). Simultaneously, White pushes Gray's left shoulder with his right hand while pulling Gray's right arm downward to the left and throwing Gray onto his back (Figure 7-61).

Key Points

a). Drop to the ground as smoothly and quickly as possible.

b). Pull the hand and push the shoulder in a circular motion to your left and coordinate it with your fall.

19. Controlling the Knee, Lifting the Waist Throw 推膝撥腰

a). Gray attempts to throw White with a hip throw (Figure 7-62).

b). White quickly squats down to prevent being thrown, gets his right hand on the front of Gray's right knee to control it, and pulls backward (Figure 7-63).

c). Simultaneously, White wraps his left arm around Gray's waist and lifts him up, then uses his body to push against Gray and make him fall forward on his face (Figure 7-64).

Key Points

a). Sink your body quickly when your opponent tries to throw you.

b). This technique is normally used to counter hip throws.

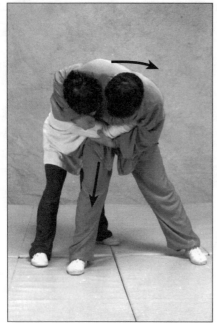

Figure 7-62

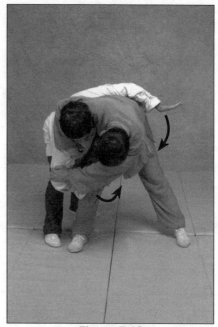

Figure 7-63

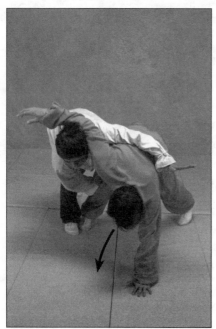

Figure 7-64

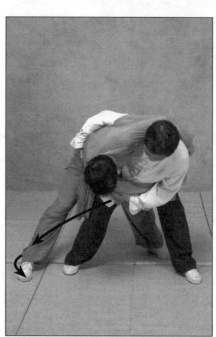

Figure 7-65

20. Controlling the Foot, Leaning Forward Throw 啃腿擠靠

a). White attempts a hip throw on Gray. Gray senses the attempt and quickly squats down to prevent the throw (Figure 7-65).

b). White switches techniques by extending his right leg and inserting it between Gray's legs. White uses his right foot to hook Gray's right ankle and uses his left hand to reach down

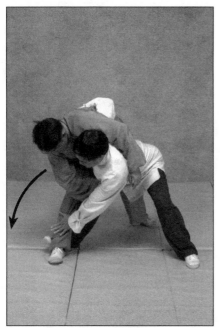
Figure 7-66

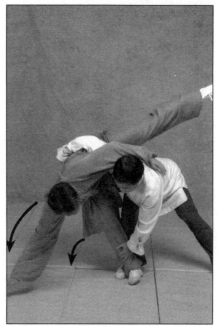
Figure 7-67

and press on Gray's foot to prevent him from pulling his leg away (Figure 7-66).

c). White leans forward and presses his right shoulder against Gray's body, still using his left hand to control the foot. White pushes forward with his left foot to make Gray fall sideways (Figure 7-67).

Key Points

a). This technique can be used as a counter to technique #19 above. It also can be used as a follow-up technique if your first throw is unsuccessful.

b). Use your back foot to push into the ground to generate more power for the takedown.

21. Pressing the Neck, Lifting the Knee Throw 壓頸托膝

a). Gray shoots in and grabs White's right leg in an attempt to throw him (Figure 7-68).

b). White immediately squats down to prevent him from executing the throw and uses his left hand to grab and push Gray's neck. Simultaneously, White steps forward into Horse Stance and uses his right hand to scoop and lift Gray's right knee (Figure 7-69).

c). White pushes Gray's neck down and continues to lift Gray's knee to flip him onto his back (Figure 7-70).

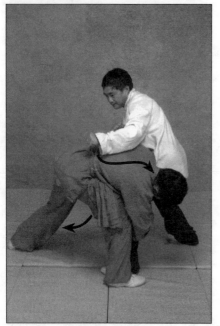

Figure 7-68

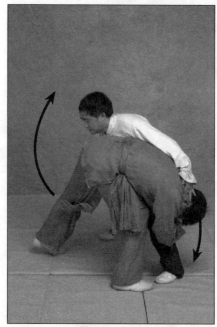

Figure 7-69

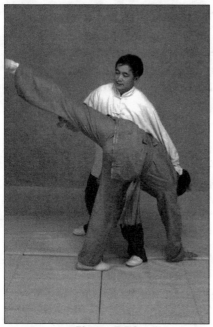

Figure 7-70

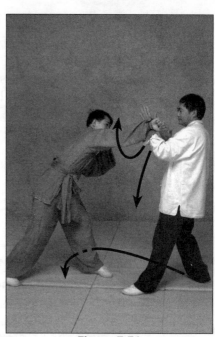

Figure 7-71

Key Points

a). The coordination of both hands is essential to the success of this technique. Your left and right hands must move simultaneously in opposite directions to create symmetry power.

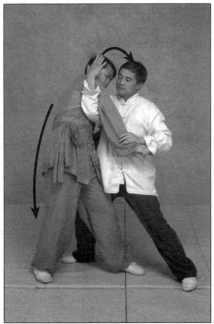

Figure 7-72

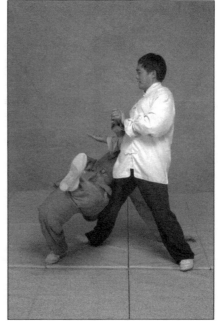

Figure 7-73

22. Lifting the Elbow, Sideways Throw 扛肘側摔

a). With his left foot forward, Gray attacks with his right hand. White moves his head to the right to avoid the punch, blocks with his left hand, and grabs Gray's wrist (Figure 7-71).

b). White steps forward with his right foot and pulls Gray's arm down close to his body. At the same time, White scoops his right arm under Gray's right armpit and lifts him up. White presses his right leg against Gray's left (Figure 7-72).

c). As White lifts and pulls, he also twists his body to the right and uses his knee to jerk upward and to the left against the back of Gray's left leg, throwing him down (Figure 7-73).

Key Points

a). The lifting and turning of your body and the use of your right leg to block should happen simultaneously.

b). Throughout the throw, keep your left leg bent for good root and balance.

23. Catching the Leg, Stepping Forward, and Shoulder Striking

Throw 撥腿上步前撞

a). Gray attacks with a right heel kick or right side kick. White uses his left hand to catch the foot and scoop upwards (Figure 7-74).

b). White then drops Gray's right leg, and before Gray can regain

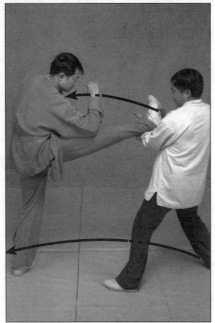

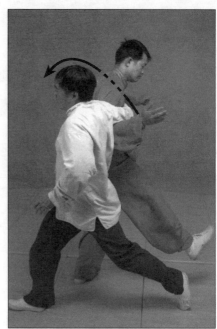

Figure 7-74   **Figure 7-75**

his balance White charges in with his right foot. Using his right arm and shoulder, White strikes Gray's chest, neck or head and pushes forward to drive Gray to the ground (Figures 7-75 and 7-76).

Key Points

a.) When catching your opponent's kick, scoop up high enough to unbalance him before dropping his foot.

b). When stepping forward, keep your knees bent for good balance.

c). Step forward as quickly as possible to create greater momentum and greater impact.

d.) Drive forward and through your opponent to complete the takedown.

24. Dropping the Body, Scissor Legs Throw

轉身高掃腿烏龍絞柱

a). White attacks with a turning back kick and Gray traps the leg (Figure 7-77).

b). White drops immediately to the ground, using both hands to break the fall. At the same time he quickly slides his left leg behind Gray's leg(s) (Figure 7-78).

c). White twists his hip clockwise and swings his left leg forward and his right leg backward to execute a scissors-like movement, and uses the turning momentum to take Gray down

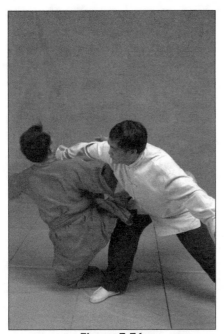

Figure 7-76

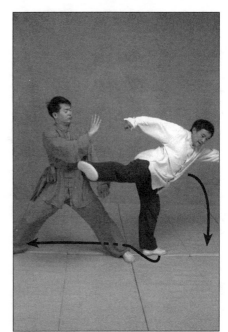

Figure 7-77

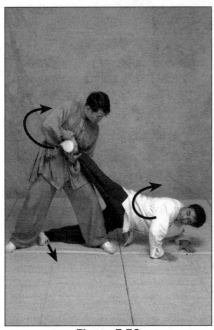

Figure 7-78

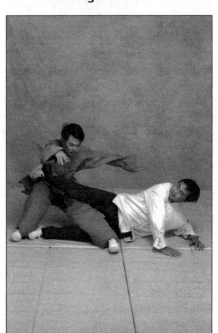

Figure 7-79

(Figure 7-79).

Key Points

a). Once your leg is trapped, drop to the ground as quickly as possible. Use both hands and arms to absorb the impact of the fall.

b). You can add more power to the takedown by pushing against

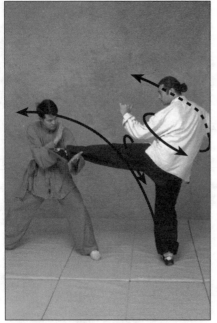

Figure 7-80

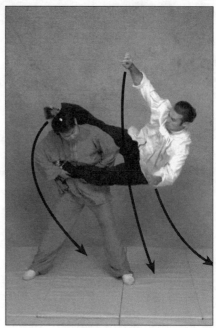

Figure 7-81

the ground and springing up slightly.

25. Leaping Up Scissor Legs Throw 騰空剪刀腳

a). White attacks with a left heel kick or side kick. Gray catches and traps the kick (Figure 7-80).

b). Using the trapped leg as a supporting point, White leaps into the air and twists his body from left to right, using the right leg to kick the back of Gray's head (Figure 7-81).

c). Simultaneously, White moves his left leg backward while continuing to kick downward with the right. Both legs make a scissors-like movement while White is still in the air. White twists counter-clockwise to generate increased momentum to bring Gray down with him. White falls with his body sideways, and uses his hands and arms to break the fall (Figure 7-82).

Key Points

a). When falling to the ground, open both hands so that your palms face the ground. The palms should make contact first, followed by the forearms. Keep both arms bent. This technique can be dangerous for both partners, so be sure to use caution when practicing.

26. Rolling Forward Throw 騰空滾壓

a). With his right foot forward, Gray attacks with his right hand. White blocks the punch with his right hand (Figure 7-83).

b). White drops low and steps forward, right foot in front, seizes

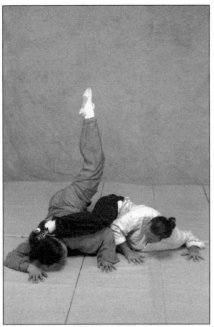

Figure 7-82

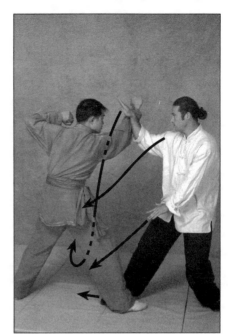

Figure 7-83

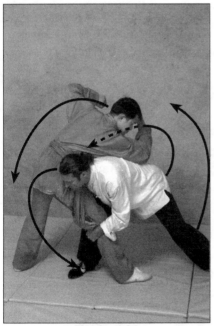

Figure 7-84

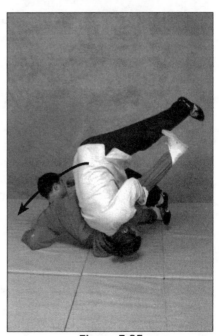

Figure 7-85

Gray's right leg with both hands, and tries to throw him. Gray detects the throw and resists (Figure 7-84).

c). White holds Gray's leg and pulls it toward his body, causing Gray to lean forward. White then dives and rolls forward, using his momentum to take Gray down. White rolls on top of Gray with his back (Figure 7-85).

Key Points

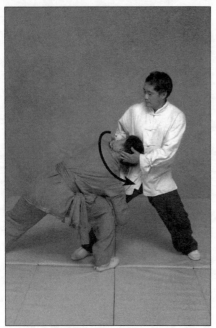

Figure 7-86

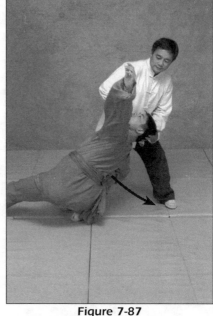

Figure 7-87

a). To land on top of your opponent, roll your body forward at a slight diagonal angle.

b). This technique relies on good tumbling skills.

27. Prevent the Leg Hold, Twist the Neck Throw
防抱腿、擰頸摔

a). Gray holds White's front leg with both hands and attempts to throw him. White sinks his weight down low to resist. White then grabs the back of Gray's head with his left hand and puts his right hand on the right side of Gray's chin (Figure 7-86).

b). White turns his body to the left and also twists Gray's head to the left to take him down. (Figure 7-87).

Key Points

a). Do not twist your partner's head sharply when practicing. This will help to prevent neck injuries.

Chapter 8
Groundfighting/Ground Controlling Techniques

地上控制法

8-1. Introduction

In many self-defense situations, groundfighting skills are just as important as standing fighting skills. You may find yourself on the ground either because of a fall or a takedown. Because the main purpose of this book is to introduce San Shou Kuai Jiao techniques for self defense, and because groundfighting is a complex subject, we will introduce only a few of the basic principles and techniques of groundfighting in this chapter.

Standing fighting and groundfighting are two very different ways of dealing with attackers. Very often a person who is well-versed in one form will lose confidence when dealing with the other. It is to your advantage to train both forms of fighting.

Generally speaking, groundfighting involves grappling with an opponent on the ground using holds, locks, and strangles. Groundfighting includes attacks and defenses from the supine position (laying on your back, or face up) and the prone position (laying on your front, or face down). A characteristic of groundfighting is a reliance on both strength and skills. Knowing the correct angle to lock or hold an opponent and being able to use your body weight to your advantage is of utmost importance. In general, the advantage of size and strength is minimized when on the ground.

While groundfighting techniques are used mostly to control an opponent and to defend against attacks while on the ground, they can also be used in standing positions. In fact, standing control techniques are more commonly used in most Chinese martial styles, and in other styles such as Jujitsu and Aikido. The term Qin Na generally represents the grap-

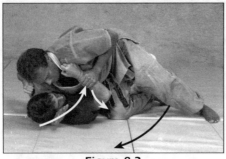

Figure 8-2

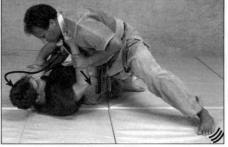

Figure 8-1

pling and controlling techniques used in almost all Chinese martial styles. The concept and principles of Qin Na are complicated and beyond the scope of this book. Readers interested in Qin Na should refer to the series of Qin Na books written by Dr. Yang, Jwing-Ming and published by YMAA. These books will give you detailed insight into this Chinese self-defense art.

As mentioned above, the art of groundfighting is complex. In this chapter, we will briefly introduce some basic groundfighting techniques. These techniques are simple and very easy to learn. Safety is extremely important when practicing these techniques with a partner. Avoid the use of excessive power during practice to help prevent injury. If you execute a technique correctly, you do not need a great deal of power to cause pain. Careless practice will result in damage to your body, perhaps even permanent damage. Let your partner know immediately when you feel pain or faintness during practice.

8-2. Groundfighting/Ground Controlling Techniques

1). Head Lock/Arm Bar 鎖頸上壓肘

a). From a supine position, Black grabs Gray's lapels with both hands. Gray, kneeling at Black's right side, slips his right arm inside Black's left arm. Gray then grabs Black's right arm with his left hand (Figure 8-1).

b). Gray collapses his weight onto Black's chest as he encircles Black's neck with his right arm while maintaining control of Black's right arm. Gray begins to slide his right leg forward (Figure 8-2).

c). Gray grabs his own lapel with his right hand to strengthen the one-arm head lock and pulls Black's arm down and across his right thigh so that his thigh is above Black's elbow for proper breaking leverage. Gray keeps his legs spread wide for maximum stability (Figure 8-3).

d). Gray leans forward and buries his head to avoid a rear-hand grab of his head or hair (Figure 8-4).

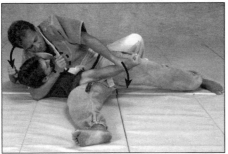

Figure 8-3

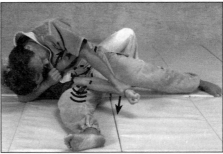

Figure 8-4

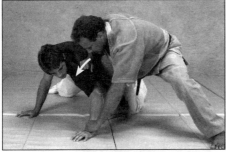

Figure 8-5

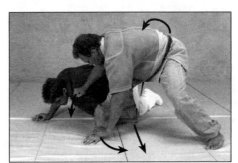

Figure 8-6

Key Points

a.) Simultaneously drop your body weight onto your opponent's chest and apply the head lock.

b.) For the straight arm bar to be most effective, your thigh must be above your opponent's elbow.

c.) Keep your weight forward to apply maximum pressure to the straight arm bar and to prevent your opponent from tipping you backwards.

2). Arm Pit Hold 腋下壓肘

a). Black is on all fours. Gray approaches him from the left side and jams his right shin against the left side of Black's torso. Gray grabs Black's left shoulder with his right arm and Black's left wrist with his left hand (Figure 8-5).

b). Gray simultaneously presses his right forearm down onto Black's left shoulder and pulls Black's left arm away from his body with the left hand. Black begins to collapse (Figure 8-6).

c). Letting go of the shoulder, Gray pulls Black's left arm up off the ground and covers it with his right armpit while twisting counterclockwise. This pins Black's face down. Gray keeps Black's left arm in a weak, elevated position with the hand palm up (Figure 8-7).

d). Gray uses both hands to apply a straight arm wrist lock to Black's left wrist. To secure the pin, Gray transfers his weight

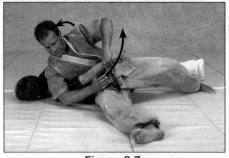

Figure 8-7

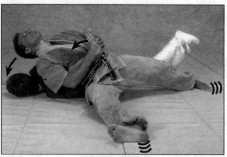

Figure 8-8

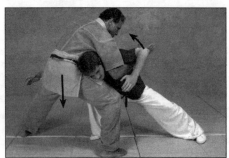

Figure 8-9

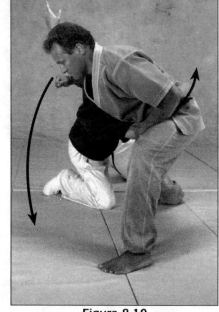

Figure 8-10

off the buttocks by bridging slightly and turning into Black's left shoulder. Finally, Gray slides his armpit down off Black's shoulder and onto his upper arm in order to apply breaking pressure to the elbow (Figure 8-8).

Key Points
a.) Keep your legs spread wide apart for stability.

3). Neck Crank 防抱腰返轉鎖頸

a). Black lunges in for a single leg takedown. Gray lowers his center of gravity, adopts a wide stance and catches Black by hooking his right arm under Black's left and hooking his left arm over Black's right (Figure 8-9).

b). Gray pivots to his left, pulling Black's right arm downwards and across the waist and raising Black's left arm and driving it behind him to flip Black onto his back (Figure 8-10).

c). Dropping onto his right knee, Gray plants his right hand on the ground while maintaining control over Black's right arm, which is across Gray's waist. Gray's left leg is out for stability (Figure 8-11).

d). Gray carefully sits through with his right leg. This weight shift causes Gray's right armpit to exert tremendous pressure on

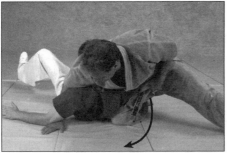

Figure 8-11

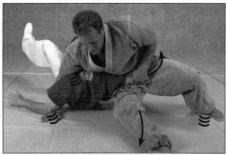

Figure 8-12

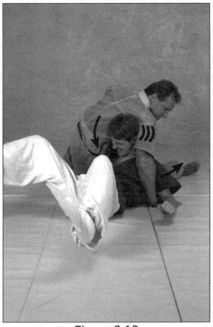

Figure 8-13

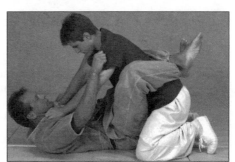

Figure 8-14

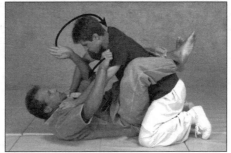

Figure 8-15

the back of Black's neck (Figure 8-12).

e). This is the rear view. Note how Gray's right arm descends to the ground across the front of Black's left shoulder and between his elbow and the left side of his body (Figure 8-13).

Key Points

a). Remember to sink low and firmly to prevent your opponent from applying the single leg takedown.

4). Reclining Guillotine 斜倚壓頸鎖喉

a). Black is in Gray's guard and attempts to choke Gray's neck. Gray buries his chin into his chest to protect his throat (Figure 8-14).

b). Gray then inserts his left arm inside Black's right arm to force the arm outward and partially break the choke (Figure 8-15).

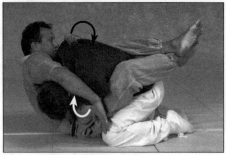
Figure 8-16

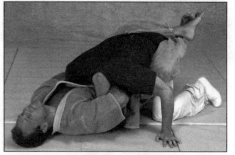
Figure 8-17

c). Gray sits up and reaches up behind Black's back with his left hand, grabbing the clothing on Black's back and pulling Black into him as he slides his right arm over Black's head. Gray now has Black in a reverse headlock with Black's neck in Gray's right armpit (Figure 8-16).

d). Gray adjusts his headlock so that the radial edge of his forearm lies across Black's throat. Next, Gray slides his left arm under Black's right armpit and between their bodies so that he can grab his left hand with his right to secure the head lock. (If Gray cannot clasp hands he will hold a piece of Black's clothing.) Then Gray pulls his right forearm up towards his head while using his legs to push Black's hips in the opposition direction, as if to stretch Black's spine. This will effectively apply excruciating pain in Black's throat (Figure 8-17).

Key Points

a.) When applying the headlock you can temporarily unhook your ankles if you experience difficulty in climbing up onto your opponent's neck. Be sure to hook the ankles after you've achieved the headlock.

b.) Use caution when pulling your partner's head and pushing his hips in opposite directions.

5). Seated Straight Arm Hug 直座摟臂

a). Black is on all fours and grabs at Gray's left leg with his left hand. Gray grabs the arm with his left hand and pulls it upward while pushing down on Black's right shoulder. This forces Black's head to the ground. Gray then steps over Black's neck with his left leg and uses his right knee to smash Black in the ribs (Figure 8-18).

b). Gray then steps over Black's head with his right leg, keeping the feet close together (Figure 8-19).

c). Gray sits backwards onto his buttocks (Figure 8-20).

d). Gray remains in a seated position, still controlling Black's left

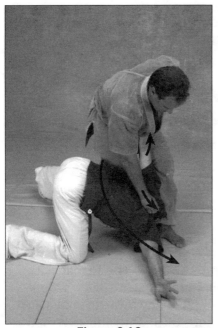

Figure 8-18

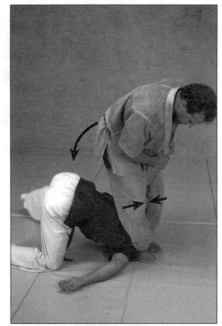

Figure 8-19

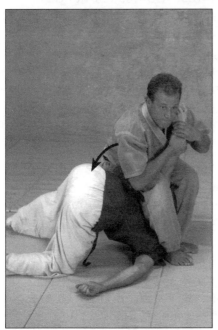

Figure 8-20

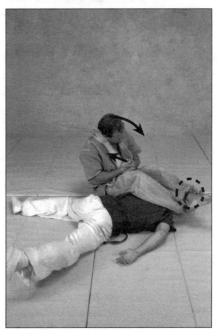

Figure 8-21

arm. The hand is palm down and pinched between Gray's right shoulder and cheek, while he cups both hands just above Black's elbow. Gray crosses his ankles and squeezes his knees together over Black's left shoulder (Figure 8-21).

Key Points

a.) Maintain control over your opponent's straight left arm with both of your hands and by squeezing your legs together.

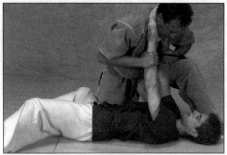

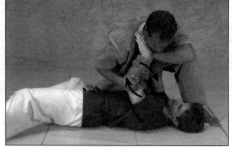

Figure 8-22   Figure 8-23

b.) After sitting back onto your buttocks, keep your torso upright.

6). Upward Arm Wrap 上纏肘

a). From a supine position Black grabs Gray by the throat with both hands. Gray, kneeling on his right leg near Black's right side, grabs Black's lower arms and pulls downward while also lifting his body to take the pressure off his neck. Gray then clears Black's right hand off his throat with his left hand and buries his chin in his chest. Gray also has the option to drop his left knee onto Black's face (Figure 8-22).

b). Gray releases Black's right arm and switches his left hand to just above the inside of Black's left wrist and slides his own right arm down to the inside of Black's left elbow. Gray drops his torso and pushes his right hand forward and right arm backwards against Black's left arm in order to bend it at the elbow (Figure 8-23).

c). Gray continues to use his left hand to push Black's left arm down towards the ground at the left side of his head while sliding his right arm along the inside of Black's left elbow until Gray can grab the top of his own left wrist (Figure 8-24).

d). Gray lies transversely across Black so that his body weight sits on Black's chest. Gray drops his left elbow to the ground, keeping Black's left wrist pinned there as he raises Black's left elbow by levering it up with his right arm. If Gray cannot obtain sufficient leverage to cause pain in Black's shoulder joint, he can roll his upper body to his left and/or draw in both arms along the ground so Black's left wrist moves closer to Black's left shoulder, maintaining downward pressure (Figure 8-25).

Key Points
a.) Protect your throat by tucking your chin to your chest.

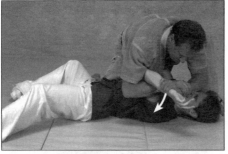

Figure 8-24

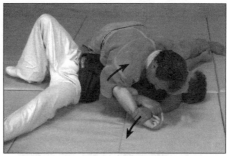

Figure 8-25

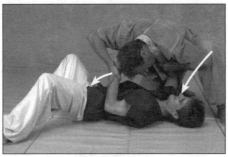

Figure 8-26

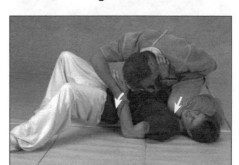

Figure 8-27

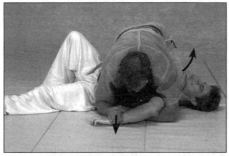

Figure 8-28

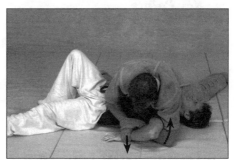

Figure 8-29

7). Downward Arm Wrap 下纏肘

a). From a supine position Black grabs Gray by the left collar with his right hand and by the hair with his left hand. Gray, kneeling on his right knee transversely to Black's right side, grabs both of Black's wrists (Figure 8-26).

b). Gray places his left knee across Black's throat and pushes down until Black releases his grip (Figure 8-27).

c). Gray pushes Black's left arm to the ground, then releases Black's right arm and wraps his left arm around the top of Black's left upper arm and between Black's left forearm and body. Gray then grabs the top of his own right wrist (Figure 8-28).

d). Gray then takes his left knee off Black's throat, shifts his weight onto Black's chest and spreads his legs wide apart for stability (Figure 8-29).

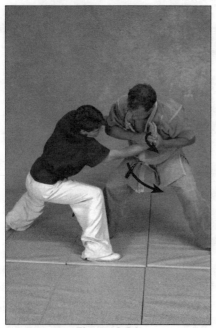

Figure 8-30

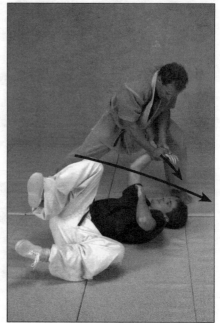

Figure 8-31

Key Points

a.) When practicing with a partner, be careful not to press your knee too forcefully into his throat.

b.) After you have shifted your weight to your opponent's chest, you can draw his captured left wrist towards his left armpit and lever his elbow off the floor with your left arm for additional torque on the shoulder.

8). Outside Wrist Lock Throw to Straight Arm Wrist Lock

Hold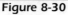

a). From a standing position Black grabs Gray's right upper arm with his left hand and Gray's left lapel with his right hand. Gray grabs Black's right hand with both of his so that Gray's thumbs go down the back of Black's wrist toward his fingers. Gray then drops into a deeper stance and rotates his hips and upper body counter-clockwise to the left (Figure 8-30).

b). Gray continues the rotation, keeping Black's arm bent at a 90 degree angle until Black flips onto his back (Figure 8-31).

c). Using the momentum of the flip, Gray rolls Black over onto his stomach and straightens his arm. Gray takes a cross step with his right foot over the top of Black's head. Gray keeps Black's fingers pointed at his head during this roll by rotating Black's hand, palm down, in a clockwise direction (Figure 8-32).

d). Gray applies a Straight Arm Wrist Lock, pushes down on Black's hand, and drops his right knee at a 45 degree angle

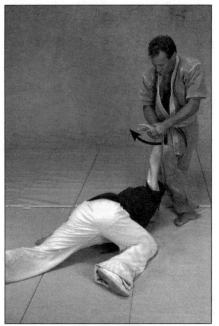

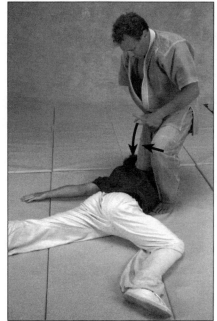

Figure 8-32   Figure 8-33

across Black's shoulder blades to further secure him. Gray can also use both knees to squeeze Black's arm above and below his elbow joint to apply pressure to the elbow (Figure 8-33).

Key Points

a.) The wrist throw, flip, and cross step should happen in one fluid motion.

9). Front Shoulder Crank 前鎖肩

a). From a supine position Black grabs Gray's lapels. Kneeling on Black's left side, Gray grabs Black's left wrist with his right hand while inserting his left hand inside Black's right arm to grab Black's right lapel (Figure 8-34).

b). Gray transfers his weight forward and then presses down on Black with his left arm and steps over Black's head with his right leg, chopping Black on the left side of the neck as he steps. This is to distract Black and help loosen his right hand grip on Gray's lapel, which Gray removes with an outward push of his left arm (Figure 8-35).

c). Gray then draws his right heel forcefully into Black's neck to keep Black from spinning out counter-clockwise. Maintaining his grip on Black's left wrist with his right hand, Gray takes his left hand and grabs the blade of Black's left hand in order twist the arm counter-clockwise. Gray slides his right arm down Black's left forearm to bend it at the elbow, pulling it counter-

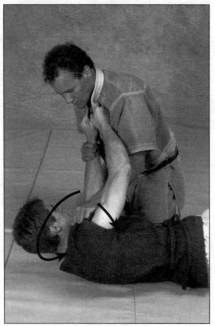

Figure 8-34

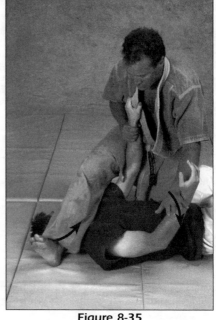

Figure 8-35

clockwise across his stomach as he does so (Figure 8-36).

d). Gray then snakes his left arm under Black's forearm and grabs his own right wrist, maintaining the positive torque on Black's arm. Black's left arm is now bent 90 degrees, with his wrist slightly lower than his forearm. Gray twists his upper body counter-clockwise to apply an extremely painful Front Shoulder Crank (Figure 8-37).

Key Points

a.) Use your right heel to ensure that your opponent can't twist out of your hold.

10). Rear Shoulder Crank 后锁肩

a). Black, from a supine position, grabs Gray's lapels. Kneeling on Black's left side, Gray grabs Black's wrists to break the grip (Figure 8-38).

b). Ignoring Black's left hand, Gray hooks his right arm under Black's right elbow and lifts upward while pushing downward on Black's right wrist, stepping up onto his left knee as he does so. This gives Gray enough lifting power to roll Black onto his left side. Gray then steps his left leg over Black's torso so that the foot is tight against Black's lower back. Black now cannot spin out of Gray's hold (Figure 8-39).

c). Gray slips his right hand out and then back over the top of Black's right upper arm, under Black's forearm and near the elbow. Black's arm is now bent at a right angle (Figure 8-40).

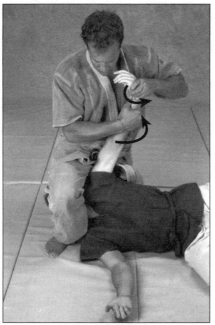

Figure 8-36

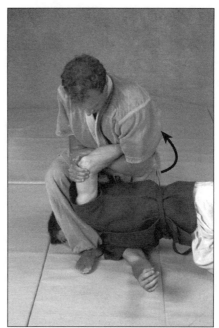

Figure 8-37

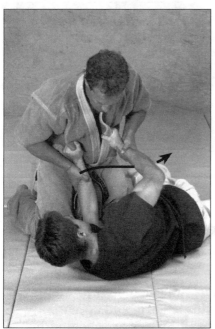

Figure 8-38

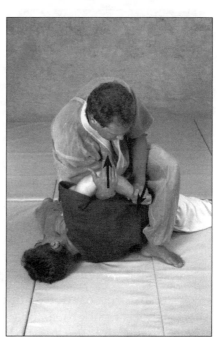

Figure 8-39

d). Gray grabs the top of his own left wrist with his right hand and turns his upper body to the right in a clockwise direction to apply the Rear Shoulder Crank (Figure 8-41).

Key Points

a.) Be sure your opponent cannot roll out of your hold.

b.) After grabbing your own wrist to apply the Shoulder Crank, your opponent's wrist should be slightly lower than his forearm.

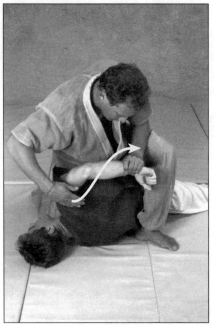

Figure 8-40

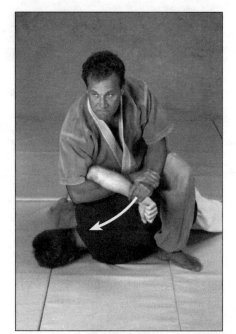

Figure 8-41

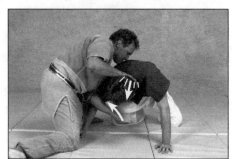

Figure 8-42

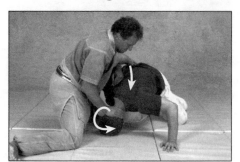

Figure 8-43

11). Turkey Wing Hold 右反肩鎖頸

a). Black is on all fours. Gray approaches from Black's right front quarter and drops to his right knee. Gray slaps the back of Black's neck with his right hand to distract Black, and hooks his left arm under Black's right arm at the elbow (Figure 8-42).

b). Gray presses downward on Black's neck and upward on Black's right arm as Gray torques his left arm and upper body clockwise to his left in order to bend Black's arm behind his back (Figure 8-43).

c). Next, Gray encircles Black's throat with his right arm by sliding it under Black's jaw (Figure 8-44).

d). Sitting backwards, Gray pulls Black close as he clasps his hands together. To complete the hold, Gray squeezes the sides of Black's neck with his right arm while pulling Black's right forearm away from his back. Black is now simultaneous-

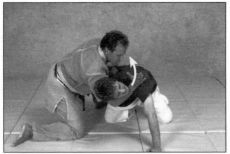

Figure 8-44

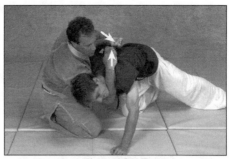

Figure 8-45

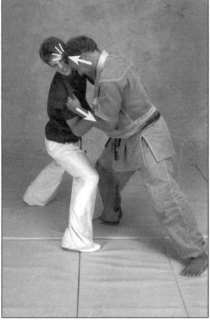

Figure 8-46

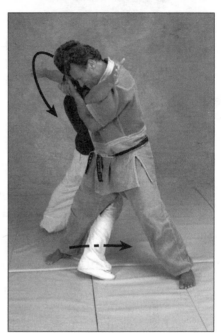

Figure 8-47

ly in a Lateral Vascular Neck Restraint hold and an opposite side Hammer Lock, called the Turkey Wing (Figure 8-45).

Key Points

a). After clasping your hands together, you may lever against your opponent's throat, turning counter-clockwise to your left and laying backwards, taking him into a Reverse Guard Position.

12). Shoulder Hold 鎖肩

a). Black and Gray seize each other's clothes. Gray pulls Black close and headbutts Black with the front portion of his skull (Figure 8-46).

b). While Black is dazed, Gray slides his right arm around the left side of Black's neck and his left arm under Black's right armpit and clasps his hands together. At the same time, Gray steps his right leg behind Black's right (Figure 8-47).

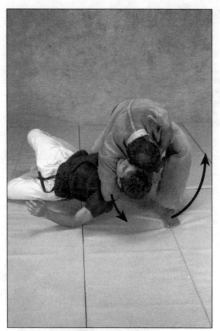

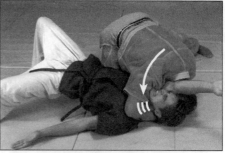

Figure 8-49

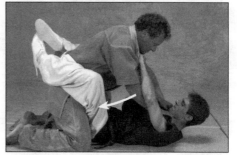

Figure 8-48

Figure 8-50

c). Gray twists his hips and upper body counter-clockwise to the left to unbalance Black, then sweeps his right leg backwards to knock Black backwards. Taking Black to the ground, Gray drops on his right knee and presses it into the left side of Black's body (Figure 8-48).

d). Gray unlocks his hands and uses his left hand to push Black's right upper arm over to the right side of his neck as he outrigs his left leg for stability. Gray then re-clasps his hands to secure Black's right arm and neck. Dropping his upper torso to the ground, Gray presses his head into Black's. Gray keeps his right elbow on the ground, using his whole body weight to pinch Black's neck between his right upper and right lower arm (Figure 8-49).

Key Points

a.) Use caution when practicing the head butt as you can seriously injure both your partner and yourself.

b.) Wrapping your opponent around the neck and armpit and stepping your leg behind his should be smooth and quick.

13). Elbow Escape from the Front Guard 擺脫鎖腰頭撞

a). Black has Gray in the Front Guard Position and both have grabbed each other's lapels (Figure 8-50).

b). Gray uses his right elbow to gouge the inside of Black's thigh and presses downwards and outwards (Figure 8-51).

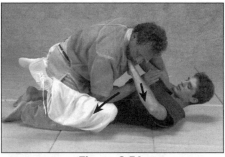

Figure 8-51

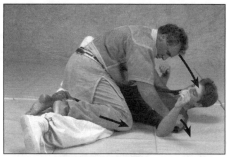

Figure 8-52

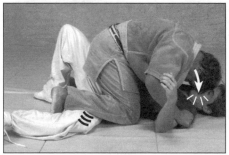

Figure 8-53

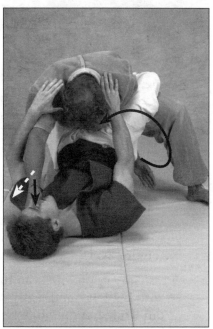

Figure 8-54

c). As he presses Black's left leg down, Gray shifts his right knee over Black's inner thigh, then pins it to the ground with his shin as his knee slides over the top of Black's leg and down to the ground. Gray then pushes Black's left arm away from him and pins it to the ground as well (Figure 8-52).

d). Gray climbs over Black's right leg with his left knee, pins Black's other arm to the floor and headbutts Black with the top front portion of his skull (Figure 8-53).

Key Points

a.) You must replace your elbow with your knee as quickly as possible to prevent your opponent from regaining his hold.

14). Turn-Over Escape from the Front Guard 反轉擺脫鎖腰

a). Black has Gray in the Front Guard and attempts to choke Gray with both hands. Gray jams the fingers of his right hand into Black's face to distract him and rises up off of his left knee and leans backward to create space between his left hip and Black's right upper thigh. Gray inserts his left arm in the opening and hooks it around the underside of Black's right leg (Figure 8-54).

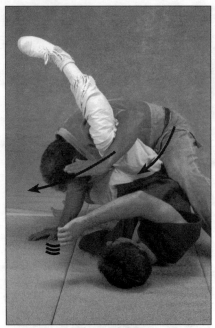

Figure 8-55

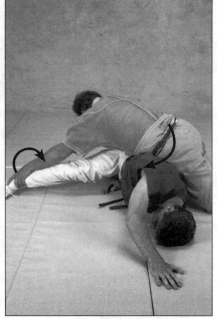

Figure 8-56

b). Gray then pushes off to the right with his left leg, planting his right hand on the ground beside Black's hip and raising his left arm, hooking Black at the knee. Gray uses his whole body to lift Black's right leg and turn him over counter-clockwise (Figure 8-55).

c). As Gray completes the turn-over, he grabs Black's right ankle with his left hand. Gray rolls onto Black's back to flatten him out while bending Black's right lower leg backwards (Figure 8-56).

d). Gray completes his roll by delivering an elbow strike to Black's head and bending Black's right leg at the knee (Figure 8-57).

Key Points

a.) After leaning back to create space between your hip and your opponent's thigh, insert your left arm up to the elbow for maximum lifting power.

b.) When you complete your roll, keep your body weight on your opponent and not on your buttocks.

15). Outside Wrist Lock Escape from the Front Mount

擺脫鎖喉外壓腕

a). Black has Gray in the Front Mount Position and tries to choke him with both hands. Gray attempts to buck Black over his head but Black is seated too high on Gray's chest and has hooked Gray's upper thighs with both feet (Figure 8-58).

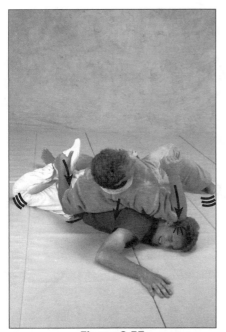

Figure 8-57

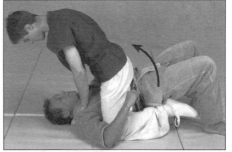

Figure 8-58

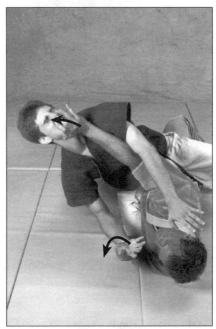

Figure 8-60

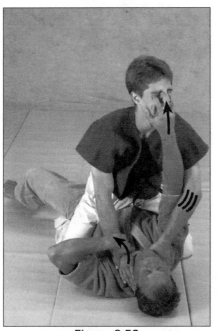

Figure 8-59

b). Gray grabs the back of Black's right hand with his left hand so that his thumb runs down the back of Black's hand and his fingers wrap around the base of Black's thumb at the palm. At the same time, Gray reaches upward inside Black's left arm and sticks his fingers into Black's eyes or pushes Black's chin away to his left (Figure 8-59).

c). Gray draws his left foot to the outside of Black's right ankle and peels Black's right wrist off his lapel with his left hand as Black reacts to the distraction. Gray twists Black's right wrist outwards in a counter-clockwise direction as he pushes off his right leg and bridges to the left (Figure 8-60).

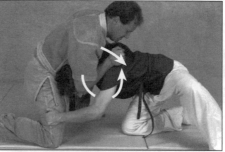

Figure 8-62

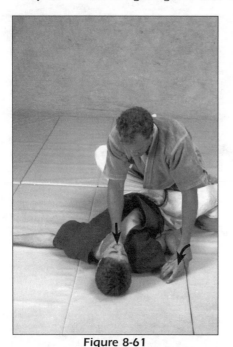

Figure 8-61

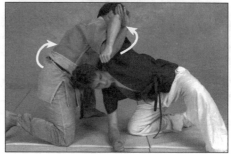

Figure 8-63

d). Gray rolls over into Black's guard, maintaining the Outside Wrist Lock. Gray finishes the technique by grabbing Black's throat with his right hand (Figure 8-61).

Key Points

a). The distraction technique (either poking the eyes or pushing the chin) is necessary to the success of this escape.

16). Roll-Over Transverse Arm Bar 返轉橫向壓肘

a). Black tackles Gray below the waist. Gray leans forward, drops onto his right knee and forces Black to the ground by jamming his right forearm into Black's left shoulder to keep Black from applying a bear hug (Figure 8-62).

b). Gray inserts his right arm under Black's left arm and hooks it up and over counter-clockwise. Simultaneously, Gray uses his left hand to push down on Black's right shoulder to spin him onto his back (Figure 8-63).

c). Gray pivots 90 degrees to the right and reclines onto his back, keeping his left leg bent to prevent Black from rolling into him. Gray covers Black's head with his right leg while maintaining control of Black's left arm (Figure 8-64).

d). Gray holds Black's head down with his right leg and squeezes his knees together. If this hurts Gray's groin, he can lever against his upper thigh by rotating his hips in the opposite direction (Figure 8-65).

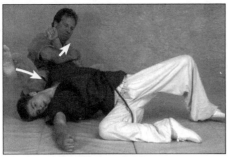

Figure 8-64

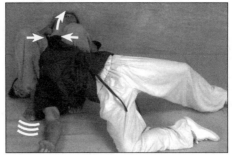

Figure 8-65

Key Points

a.) Make sure you pull your opponent's shoulder in tight to your groin and arch your back to get proper leverage as you straighten his left arm.

b.) You can turn your opponent's hand thumb up to place it in a weaker position.

Appendix A
Names of San Shou Kuai Jiao Techniques

Chapter 4—Holding Leg(s) Throws 抱腳摔

1. Holding Two Legs, Pressing Forward Throw　抱兩腿前頂摔
2. Holding One Leg, Hand Blocking Throw　抱單腿手別
3. Holding One Leg, Leg Blocking Throw　抱單腿別腿
4. Holding One Leg, Rotating the Body, Elbow Pressing Throw　摟腿旋身肘壓
5. Holding One Leg, Moving Forward and Pressing Down Throw　摟腿前按摔
6. Holding Two Legs, Sideways Throw　抱雙腿側摔
7. Holding Two Legs, Backward Throw　抱雙腿向后摔
8. Holding Two Legs, Back Falling and Turn Over Throw　抱雙腿后倒翻身摔
9. Holding and Penetrating Two Legs　抱雙腿黑狗鑽襠
10. Holding One Leg, Inner Sweeping Throw　抱單腿打腿
11. Holding One Leg, Pushing the Chest Throw　抱單腿推胸摔
12. Holding One Leg, Sideways Throw　抱單腿側拌
13. Holding One Leg, Backward Over the Shoulder Throw　抱單腿后摔
14. Holding One Leg, Lifting Up Throw　抱單腿上托
15. Holding One Leg, Pulling Throw　抱單腿下拉
16. Holding One Leg, Pressing the Neck Throw　抱單腿壓頸勾腿
17. Holding One Leg, Hooking and Pushing Forward Throw　抱單腿摟踢前推
18. Holding One Leg, Carrying Over the Shoulder Throw　抱單腿過背
19. Scooping the Leg, Shoulder Pressing Throw　抄腿掀靠
20. Holding the Leg, Pushing the Shoulder Throw　摟腿推胸
21. Holding and Checking Leg Throw　摟腿挫壓

Chapter 5—Over the Back/Holding the Waist Throws 過背抱腰摔

Over the Back Throwing Methods 過背摔法

1. Squeezing the Neck, Hip Throw 夾脖揹摔
2. Lifting the Arm, Holding the Shoulder, Over the Back Throw 插腋抱肩過背摔
3. Holding the Waist, Over the Back Throw 抱腰過背摔
4. Penetrating and Holding the Arm, Over the Back Throw 穿臂抱臂過背摔
5. Squeezing the Neck, Sweeping the Leg, Over the Back Throw 夾頸向后打腿過背摔
6. Lifting the Arm, Holding the Shoulder, Sweeping the Leg, Over the Back Throw 插腋抱肩向后打腿過背摔

Holding the Waist Throwing Methods 抱腰摔法

1. Holding the Waist, Falling Back and Turning Over Throw 抱腰后倒翻身摔
2. Holding the Waist From Behind Throw 后抱腰摔
3. Holding the Waist From Behind, Falling Backward Throw 后抱腰后倒翻身摔
4. Holding the Waist, Winding the Leg, Pressing Forward Throw 抱腰盤腿前壓
5. Strangle the Waist, Leap Up, and Strike with Head Throw 砸腰跳起頭撞摔
6. Holding the Waist, Pushing the Chin and Rotating the Body Throw 抱腰推頤旋身摔

Chapter 6—Leg Hooking Throws 勾腳摔

1. Lifting the Elbow, Hooking the Ankle Throw 扛肘摔
2. Seizing the Upper Arm, Leg Hooking Throw 拿臂撮摔
3. Picking Up the Leg Throw 撿腿摔(勾)
4. Hooking the Leg Throw 勾帶腳
5. Hook Kicking, Leg Sweeping Throw 勾踢毂腳腿
6. Lower Inner Hooking Throw 小得合
7. Hook Kicking, Lower Inner Hooking Throw 勾踢小得合
8. Pulling the Neck, Hook Kicking Throw 拔頸勾踢
9. Outside Suspending the Leg Hooking Throw 外勾挂
10. Pulling, Hook Kicking Throw 扯拉勾踢
11. Chopping, Hook Kicking Throw 劈掌勾踢
12. Holding the Leg, Chopping the Neck and Hook Kicking Throw 摟腿劈掌勾踢
13. Lifting the Elbow, Hooking Sideways Throw 扛肘勾踢
14. Suspending the Leg Hook, Striking the Back Throw 勾掛砸背
15. Suspending the Leg Hook, Pushing the Shoulder Throw 勾挂擠靠
16. Dodging, Hooking the Leg, and Pushing Throw 閃身勾挂擠靠
17. Hooking the Front and Sweeping the Back Throw 前勾后掃

Chapter 7—Other Throwing Methods 其他摔法

1. Hand Blocking, Sideways Throw 手別側摔
2. Hand Blocking, Moving Forward Throw 手別前進摔
3. Crossing Elbow Strike, Pressing the Neck Throw 橫肘頂摔

4. Moving Forward, Cutting the Neck Throw 上步切摔

5. Scooping the Groin, Crossing Back Throw 挑襠過背摔

6. Stomach Throw 倒地拉臂蹬腹過頂摔

7. Pulling the Leg, Pressing Forward Throw 拉腳前推

8. Dodging, Scooping the Groin, Pressing the Neck Throw 閃身掏襠按頸

9. Controlling the Leg and Pushing the Chest Throw 躍步管腳攔胸

10. Surrounding the Neck, Pulling Backward Throw 圈頸后拉

11. Flipping Over Throw 提翻

12. Brushing the Neck, Blocking the Knee Throw 抹脖攔膝摔

13. Twisting the Neck Throw 搓頸摔

14. Sweeping the Leg Throw 殼腳腿

15. Penetrating the Legs, Pressing and Rolling Sideways Throw
    鑽襠滾壓

16. Leaping and Pushing Forward Throw 虎扑前推

17. Penetrating the Legs, Leaning Against the Body Throw 穿腿靠

18. Falling Sideways, Pushing the Shoulder Throw 側倒推肩

19. Controlling the Knee, Lifting the Waist Throw 推膝撥腰

20. Controlling the Foot, Leaning Forward Throw 嘈腿擠靠

21. Pressing the Neck, Lifting the Knee Throw 壓頸托膝

22. Lifting the Elbow, Sideways Throw 扛肘側摔

23. Catching the Leg, Stepping Forward, and Shoulder Striking Throw
    撥腿上步前撞

24. Dropping the Body, Scissor Legs Throw 轉身高掃腿烏龍絞柱

25. Leaping Up Scissor Legs Throw 騰空剪刀腳

26. Rolling Forward Throw 騰空滾壓

27. Prevent the Leg Hold, Twist the Neck Throw 防抱腿、擰頸摔

Chapter 8—Groundfighting/Ground Controlling Techniques 地上控制法

1. Head Lock/Arm Bar 鎖頸上壓肘

2. Arm Pit Hold 腋下壓肘

3. Neck Crank 防抱腰返轉鎖頸

4. Reclining Guillotine 斜倚壓頸鎖喉

5. Seated Straight Arm Hug 直座摟臂

6. Upward Arm Wrap 上纏肘

7. Downward Arm Wrap 下纏肘

8. Outside Wrist Lock Throw to Straight Arm Wrist Lock Hold 直臂下壓腕

9. Front Shoulder Crank 前鎖肩

10. Rear Shoulder Crank 后鎖肩

11. Turkey Wing Hold 右反肩鎖頸

12. Shoulder Hold 鎖肩

13. Elbow Escape from the Front Guard 擺脫鎖腰頭撞

14. Turn-Over Escape from the Front Guard 反轉擺脫鎖腰

15. Outside Wrist Lock Escape from the Front Mount
    擺脫鎖喉外壓腕

16. Roll-Over Transverse Arm Bar 返轉橫向壓肘

Appendix B
Translation and Glossary of Chinese Terms

Aikido 合氣道
A style of Japanese martial arts which uses the same theory of Chinese Taijiquan and Qin Na.

Baguazhang 八卦掌
Means "Eight Trigram Palms." A Chinese internal martial arts style.

Bao Fa Jin 爆發勁
Literally "Explosive." A sudden, short and strong type of martial power.

Beijing 北京
Capital of China.

Beng Jin 朔勁
An extending/stretching type of martial power.

Bu 步
Stepping.

Bu Fa 步法
Generally refers to the stepping techniques or footwork used in martial arts.

Cang Zhou 滄州
Name of a city in Hebei Province, China.

Chen style Taijiquan 陳氏太極拳
One of the major styles of Taijiquan, originating from the Chen family.

Chen Village 陳家溝
The village where Chen style Taijiquan was developed.

Chen, Yuan -Yun 陳元贇
A Chinese martial artist and army officer from the Ming dynasty (1368-1644 A.D.) who is credited with influencing the arts of Jujitsu and Judo in Japan.

Chongqian 重慶
Name of a city in Sichuan province, China.

Chuan Tong Shuai Jiao 傳統摔跤
Traditional Chinese wrestling.

Chuo Jiao 戳腳
A style of Chinese martial arts which specializes in leg techniques.

Cun Bu 寸步
Inch stepping. A stepping method used in Xingyiquan.

Cun Jin 寸勁
Sometimes referred to as "Inch Power". A method used to emit power at very close range in the martial arts.

Da 打
To strike. Normally, to attack with the palms, fists or arms.

Da Peng Qigong 大鵬氣功
Literally "Great Roc Qigong." A style of Qigong developed on Emei mountain, Sichuan, China.

Emei Mountain 峨嵋山
A well-known mountain located in Sichuan province, China.

Fa 法
Martial arts method or technique.

Fujian 福建
A province located in southeast China.

Gong (Kung) 功
Energy or hard work.

Gongfu (Kung Fu) 功夫
Literally "Energy-Time." Anything which takes time and energy to learn or to accomplish is called Gongfu.

Henan 河南
A province in China. The most famous Shaolin temple is located in Henan province.

Hua Mountain 華山
A well-known mountain in Shanxi province, China.

Hua Quan Xiu Tui 花拳繡腿
Literally "Flower Fist and Brocade Leg." Generally refers to martial techniques that look nice but are not very effective.

Huang Ti 黃帝
Yellow Emperor, 2697 B.C.

Hubei 湖北
Literally "Lake North." A province in China.

Ji Bu 疾步
Urgent stepping. A stepping method used in Xingyiquan.

Ji Fa 技法
Fighting techniques and strategies used in martial arts.

Jin 勁
Martial power. A combination of "Li" (muscular power) and "Qi."

Jing 精
Essence. One of the three treasures (Jing, Qi, and Shen) in the human body.

Jing-Shen 精神
Literally "Spirit" or "Essence-Spirit." Generally translated as "Spirit of Vitality."

Judo 柔道

A style of Japanese martial arts with origins in Chinese wrestling. A modern form of Jujitsu.

Jujitsu 柔術道
A style of Japanese martial arts. It is believed that this art has been influenced by Chinese wrestling and Qin Na.

Karate 空手道
Literally, "Barehanded Way." A Japanese martial art rooted in Chinese southern White Crane style.

Kuai Jiao 快跤
Literally "Fast Wrestling."

Lei Tai 擂臺
A 24 by 24 foot platform five feet off the ground used for martial arts sparring competitions.

Li 力
The power generated from muscular strength.

Lian Jing Hua Qi 練精化氣
"To refine the Essence and convert it to Qi." A Qigong training process through which you convert Essence into Qi.

Liang Qiang Xiang Yu; Yong Zhe Sheng 兩強相遇，勇者勝
"When two strong fighters meet,the braver one will win."

Liangong Shr Ba Fa 練功十八法
Eighteen methods of Qigong training.

Liu He Ba Fa 六合八法
A Chinese internal martial art. Its techniques are combined from Taijiquan, Xingyi, and Baguazhang.

Ming 明
Ming dynasty (1368-1644 A.D.).

Na 拿
Means to hold or to grab.

Ning Jin 擰勁
The twisting type of martial power used in martial arts techniques.

Nisei Karate-do
A branch of Japanese Karate.

Qi 氣
Chinese term for universal energy. A current popular model states that the Qi circulating in the human body is bio-electricity.

Qiao 巧
Skillful or ingenious.

Qiao Jin 巧勁
Martial power applied in techniques skillfully or ingeniously.

Qigong 氣功
The Gongfu of Qi, which means the study of Qi.

Qin Na (Chin Na) 擒拿
Literally "Grab control." A component of Chinese martial arts which emphasizes grabbing techniques to control an opponent's joints in conjunction with attacking certain acupuncture cavities.

Qingchen Mountain 青城山
A well-known mountain located in Sichuan province, China.

San Bao 三寶
Three treasures. Essence (Jing), energy (Qi) and spirit (Shen). Also call San Yuan (three origins).

San Shou 散手
Literally "Random Hands." Implies techniques executed randomly, as in free fighting.

San Shou Kuai Jiao 散手快跤
Fast wrestling for free fighting.

Shanghai 上海
China's largest city located in the eastern part of the country.

Shaolin 少林
Literally "Young Woods." The name of the Shaolin Temple.

Shen 身
Body.

Shen 神
Mind or Spirit.

Shen Fa 身法
Method of body movements practiced in martial arts.

Shi Ji 時機
Opportunity. Generally refers to opportunity in fighting.

Shou 手
Hand.

Shou Fa 手法
Generally refers to hand techniques used for attack or defense in martial arts.

Shuai 摔
Literally "Throw." An abbreviation of "Shuai Jiao."

Shuai Jiao 摔跤
Chinese wrestling. Part of Chinese martial arts.

Sichuan 四川
A province in Southwestern China.

Song 宋
Song dynasty (960-1279 A D).

Su Du 速度
Speed. Refers to the speed of martial techniques.

Taiji Bu 太極步
The stepping techniques or footwork used in Taijiquan.

Taijiquan (Tai Chi Chuan) 太極拳
A Chinese internal martial art based on the theory of Taiji (grand ultimate).

Tang Ni Bu 蹚泥步
Literally "Muddy Stepping." The way that a Baguazhang practitioner walks in training.

Teinstin 天津
A city in Hebei province, China.

Ti 踢
Literally "To kick."

Tong Jin 捅勁
Thrusting power. A method of applying martial power in Chinese wrestling.

White Crane style (Bai He Quan) 白鶴拳
A Chinese southern martial arts style.

Wudang Mountain 武當山
A mountain located in Hubei province, China.

Wushu 武術
Literally " Martial techniques."

Xia Dan Tian 下丹田
Lower Dan Tian. Located in the lower abdomen, it is believed to be the residence of water Qi (Original Qi) in Qigong theory.

Xian 西安
A city located in Shanxi province, China.

Xin Li Juang Tai 心理狀態
The mental and emotional states of mind.

Xingyi 形意
An abbreviation of Xingyiquan. One of the well-known Chinese internal martial styles created by Marshal Yue Fei (1103-1142 A.D.) during the Song dynasty in China.

Yan 眼
Eye.

Yan Dao, Shou Dao, Shen Bu Ye Dao 眼到、手到、身步也到
"Eyes arrive; hands arrive; body and stepping also arrive." A summary of body coordination that is emphasized in martial arts training.

Yan Fa 眼法
Techniques of the eyes.

Yan Si Shan Dian; Shou Si Jian; Yao Si Pan She; Jiao Si Zuan
眼似閃電，手似箭。腰似盤蛇，腳似鑽。
"Eyes like lightning; hands like an arrow; waist like a coiling snake; legs like a drill." A summary of the skills emphasized in Chinese wrestling training.

Yang 陽
The positive side of the two poles. Opposite of Yin.

Yi Dan, Er Li, San Gongfu 一膽、二力、三功夫
"First, bravery; second, power; third, technique." A summary of important elements in martial arts when facing an opponent.

Yi Li Jiang Shi Hui 一力降十會
"One power suppresses ten techniques." It means power is more important than techniques.

Yin 陰
The negative side of the two poles. Opposite of Yang.

Zhan Shu 戰術
Fighting strategy.

Zuan Bu 躦步
Drill stepping. A stepping method from Xingyiquan training.

Bibliography

Du Zhong-Xun. *Shi Yong Bo Ji Shuai Fa.* Beijing Athletic Institute Publications, 1993.

Emei Shan Da Shu. Sichuan Scientific Technical Publications, 1985.

Jiang, Bai Long. *Tu Shou Ji Ji Shu.* Hunan Scientific Technical Publications, 1987.

Kang, Ge-Wu. *Zhong Guo Wushu Shi Yong Da Quan.* Today's China Publications, 1990.

Kazuzo Kudo. *Dynamic Judo: Grappling Techniques.* Japan Publications Trading Company, 1967.

Kiyoshi Kobayashi and Harold E. Sharp. *The Sport of Judo.* Charles E. Tuttle Company, 1956.

Shan Shou Yun Dong. China People's Police College Publications, 1988.

Shi Yong Fang Shen Mi Shu. Beijing Athletic Institute Publications, 1992.

Lebell, Gene. *Pro-wrestling Finishing Holds.* Pro-Action Publishing, 1985.

Dr. Yang Jwing-Ming. *Analysis of Shaolin Chin Na.* YMAA Publication Center, 1987.

Liang Shou-Yu and Dr. Yang Jwing-Ming. *Hsing Yi Chuan.* YMAA Publication Center, 1990.

Zhong Guo Shuai Shu. People's Athletic Publications, 1985.

Zhong Hua Bo Ji Shu. Beijing Athletic Institute Publications, 1993.

Zhong Guo Shan Shou. People's Athletic Publications, 1990.

Index

BOOKS FROM YMAA

VIDEOS FROM YMAA

more products available from...
YMAA Publication Center, Inc. 楊氏東方文化出版中心
4354 Washington Street Roslindale, MA 02131
1-800-669-8892 • ymaa@aol.com • www.ymaa.com

VIDEOS FROM YMAA (CONTINUED)

DEFEND YOURSELF 1 — UNARMED	T010/343
DEFEND YOURSELF 2 — KNIFE	T011/351
EMEI BAGUAZHANG 1	T017/280
EMEI BAGUAZHANG 2	T018/299
EMEI BAGUAZHANG 3	T019/302
EIGHT SIMPLE QIGONG EXERCISES FOR HEALTH 2ND ED.	T005/54X
ESSENCE OF TAIJI QIGONG	T006/238
MUGAI RYU	T050/467
NORTHERN SHAOLIN SWORD — SAN CAI JIAN & ITS APPLICATIONS	T035/051
NORTHERN SHAOLIN SWORD — KUN WU JIAN & ITS APPLICATIONS	T036/06X
NORTHERN SHAOLIN SWORD — QI MEN JIAN & ITS APPLICATIONS	T037/078
QIGONG: 15 MINUTES TO HEALTH	T042/140
SCIENTIFIC FOUNDATION OF CHINESE QIGONG — LECTURE	T029/590
SHAOLIN KUNG FU BASIC TRAINING — 1	T057/0045
SHAOLIN KUNG FU BASIC TRAINING — 2	T058/0053
SHAOLIN LONG FIST KUNG FU — TWELVE TAN TUI	T043/159
SHAOLIN LONG FIST KUNG FU — LIEN BU CHUAN	T002/19X
SHAOLIN LONG FIST KUNG FU — GUNG LI CHUAN	T003/203
SHAOLIN LONG FIST KUNG FU — YI LU MEI FU & ER LU MAI FU	T014/256
SHAOLIN LONG FIST KUNG FU — SHI ZI TANG	T015/264
SHAOLIN LONG FIST KUNG FU — XIAO HU YAN	T025/604
SHAOLIN WHITE CRANE GONG FU — BASIC TRAINING 1	T046/440
SHAOLIN WHITE CRANE GONG FU — BASIC TRAINING 2	T049/459
SHAOLIN WHITE CRANE GONG FU — BASIC TRAINING 3	T074/0185
SIMPLIFIED TAI CHI CHUAN — 24 & 48	T021/329
SUN STYLE TAIJIQUAN	T022/469
TAI CHI CHUAN & APPLICATIONS — 24 & 48	T024/485
TAI CHI FIGHTING SET	T078/0363
TAIJI BALL QIGONG — 1	T054/475
TAIJI BALL QIGONG — 2	T057/483
TAIJI BALL QIGONG — 3	T062/0096
TAIJI BALL QIGONG — 4	T063/010X
TAIJI CHIN NA	T016/408
TAIJI CHIN NA IN DEPTH — 1	T070/0282
TAIJI CHIN NA IN DEPTH — 2	T071/0290
TAIJI CHIN NA IN DEPTH — 3	T072/0304
TAIJI CHIN NA IN DEPTH — 4	T073/0312
TAIJI PUSHING HANDS — 1	T055/505
TAIJI PUSHING HANDS — 2	T058/513
TAIJI PUSHING HANDS — 3	T064/0134
TAIJI PUSHING HANDS — 4	T065/0142
TAIJI SABER	T053/491
TAIJI & SHAOLIN STAFF — FUNDAMENTAL TRAINING — 1	T061/0088
TAIJI & SHAOLIN STAFF — FUNDAMENTAL TRAINING — 2	T076/0347
TAIJI SWORD, CLASSICAL YANG STYLE	T031/817
TAIJI WRESTLING — 1	T079/0371
TAIJI WRESTLING — 2	T080/038X
TAIJI YIN & YANG SYMBOL STICKING HANDS–YANG TAIJI TRAINING	T056/580
TAIJI YIN & YANG SYMBOL STICKING HANDS–YIN TAIJI TRAINING	T067/0177
TAIJIQUAN, CLASSICAL YANG STYLE	T030/752
WHITE CRANE HARD QIGONG	T026/612
WHITE CRANE SOFT QIGONG	T027/620
WILD GOOSE QIGONG	T032/949
WU STYLE TAIJIQUAN	T023/477
XINGYIQUAN — 12 ANIMAL FORM	T020/310
YANG STYLE TAI CHI CHUAN AND ITS APPLICATIONS	T001/181

DVDS FROM YMAA

ANALYSIS OF SHAOLIN CHIN NA	D0231
BAGUAZHANG 1,2, & 3 —EMEI BAGUAZHANG	D0649
CHIN NA IN DEPTH COURSES 1 — 4	D602
CHIN NA IN DEPTH COURSES 5 — 8	D610
CHIN NA IN DEPTH COURSES 9 — 12	D629
EIGHT SIMPLE QIGONG EXERCISES FOR HEALTH	D0037
THE ESSENCE OF TAIJI QIGONG	D0215
QIGONG MASSAGE—FUNDAMENTAL TECHNIQUES FOR HEALTH AND RELAXATION	D0592
SHAOLIN KUNG FU FUNDAMENTAL TRAINING 1&2	D0436
SHAOLIN LONG FIST KUNG FU — BASIC SEQUENCES	D661
SHAOLIN WHITE CRANE GONG FU BASIC TRAINING 1&2	D599
SIMPLIFIED TAI CHI CHUAN	D0630
SUNRISE TAI CHI	D0274
TAI CHI FIGHTING SET—TWO PERSON MATCHING SET	D0657
TAIJI BALL QIGONG COURSES 1&2—16 CIRCLING AND 16 ROTATING PATTERNS	D0517
TAIJI PUSHING HANDS 1&2—YANG STYLE SINGLE AND DOUBLE PUSHING HANDS	D0495
TAIJIQUAN CLASSICAL YANG STYLE	D645
TAIJI SWORD, CLASSICAL YANG STYLE	D0452
WHITE CRANE HARD & SOFT QIGONG	D637

more products available from...

YMAA Publication Center, Inc.　楊氏東方文化出版中心

4354 Washington Street Roslindale, MA 02131

1-800-669-8892 • ymaa@aol.com • www.ymaa.com